The toxic consumer

About the authors

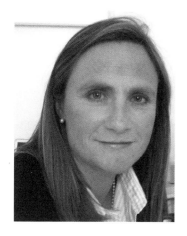

Elizabeth Salter Green is the Director of the Toxics Programme for WWF UK. Her first degree is in clinical physiology, specialising in endocrinology. This was followed by six years of marine research. Her second degree is in international environmental law. Having worked for WWF UK for ten years, Elizabeth has been Director of the European Toxics Programme for WWF International and been seconded to the UN Balkans Task Force re. pollution generated via NATO bombing. Priorities within the UK Toxics Programme are EDCs (endocrine-disrupting chemicals) and VPVBs (very persistent and very bioaccumulative chemicals). REACH (Registration, Evaluation and Authorisation of Chemicals) is a political priority and current activities include a Biomonitoring Programme.

Karen Ashton is a freelance writer and arts consultant with a background in PR and advertising. She has always been concerned about environmental issues and first became interested in the subject of toxic chemicals while researching an eco-espionage novel that featured chemical industry corruption as part of its plot. She is now committed to writing further on the subject for the non-fiction market.

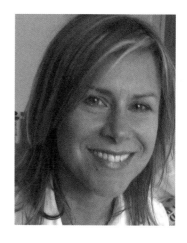

The toxic consumer

How to reduce your exposure to everyday toxic chemicals

The toxic consumer

ISBN 1 904601 42 1

First published in Great Britain in 2006 by Impact Publishing Ltd.
12 Pierrepont Street, Bath, BA1 1LA
info@impactpublishing.co.uk
www.impactpublishing.co.uk

Printing (sheet-fed litho)
Printed in the UK by the Cambrian Press who hold ISO14001 certification for environmental awareness. Inks are vegetable-based, water and solvents recycled. Files were transferred electronically with plates made direct from print resolution PDFs supplied by the publisher.

Paper
Printed on Era Silk and Tauro Offset.

Era Silk is manufactured from 50 per cent genuine waste pulp, with the balance of pulp from certified forests. The waste element contains fibres recovered from communities across the south-east of England.

Tauro Offset is ISO 14001 accredited being manufactured to high environmental standards, with a total use of energy and raw materials lower than for other types of paper. Pulp is obtained almost exclusively from thinned out and waste timber from sustainable forests close to the mill. The paper is TCF (totally chlorine free).

Foreword

It's undoubtedly true, in almost all fields of science, that the more we discover, the more we realise how much there still is to discover.

Reflecting on the astonishing progress made over the last fifty years in the development and use of chemicals throughout society, one can't help but conclude that this is an industry that would have done well to apply itself more systematically to the things it **didn't** know before rushing ahead quite so precipitately on the basis of what it **did** know to create yet more products and yet more "smart solutions".

Even now, the combined legacy effects of fifty years of unprecedented innovation in this field of science remain unclear. There are many (particularly those who still work in the chemicals industry) who are unperturbed at the fact that literally thousands of chemical compounds have been made use of during that time without any effort to test for potential impacts on the physical environment or on human health.

There are others (including the authors of this book) who are far less sanguine. It is their contention, across a very wide range of chemicals already known to be toxic, that the more evidence we gather about those impacts, the more reason we have to be very worried indeed.

This creates an almost intractable stand-off. Of all the different industries that Forum for the Future has worked with over the last decade, it is the chemicals industry that has proved most defensive and most resistant to change. With all the work we did with the now defunct Chemistry Leadership Council (with the specific intent of making the case for a far more precautionary and sustainable approach to the development and use of chemicals), it always felt as if we were working **against** the grain of an industry still disinclined to acknowledge that there are any basic flaws in its historic business model.

But the kind of bland reassurances industry experts once relied on to "manage" public concern are now completely inadequate. Consumers are becoming much more demanding, much less prepared simply to give chemical companies "the benefit of the doubt". And as consumers become less tolerant, so too do the retailers who provide for their wants and needs. What this means, in practice, is that it's the likes of Marks and Spencer and Boots, as well as industry leaders like S C Johnson, that are putting the real pressure on the industry to get its act together.

That's good news as far as Elizabeth Salter Green and the WWF UK are concerned, not least as they remain more than a little disillusioned with the way governments have so signally failed to regulate the industry properly. The latest EU regulations provide just the latest example of too little being done too late – yet again as a result of unprecedented lobbying by the industry across the whole of Europe.

To which the best response is surely for all of us to get a lot more educated about the chemicals in our lives than we are today – and that's exactly what *"The Toxic Consumer"* is all about.

– *Jonathon Porritt*

Jonathon Porritt is Founder Director of Forum for the Future, Chairman of the UK Sustainable Development Commission (www.sd-commission.org.uk) and author of a number of books including *Capitalism as If the World Matters*.

Preface

This book seeks to show that there is an increasing body of evidence pointing to a possible link between the rise of certain non-infectious human health problems and the increase in our exposure to many synthetic chemicals. We are unable to state categorically that toxic man-made chemicals are the cause of certain illnesses or are necessarily detrimental to human health because of the plethora of different factors that affect any given individual at any one time. What we do know for certain is that the widespread use of man-made chemicals in industrialised nations has led to global contamination of the environment, wildlife and humankind and that many chemicals in everyday consumer products have been found to contaminate human tissue. The presence of certain man-made chemicals at current environmental levels may well be having a negative impact on both wildlife and human health. The results of laboratory studies, case histories of accidental chemical contamination in the past, the direct measurement of chemical exposure in humans and correlative data between levels of exposure to chemicals and the incidence of certain disorders all support the wisdom of adopting a precautionary approach with regard to hazardous chemicals. This book supports the view that we should minimise our exposure to those chemicals suspected to have toxic effects until the full extent of their toxicity on human health has been determined – and where chemicals are shown to be toxic to human health, that safer alternatives should be sought.

For Florence, Frederick and Ava May

Thank you to WWF UK for their ground breaking work in the area of toxic chemicals.

To find out more go to www.wwf.org.uk

CONTENTS

Introduction

The extent to which man-made chemicals, in their comparatively short history, have become infused into the fabric of twenty first century lifestyles is astonishing. The first synthetic chemicals were created in the late 1800's, but it wasn't until post World War II that the industry really took off. Chemists previously engaged in developing chemical weapons for use in combat realised that many of the deadly poisons they had been concocting had a useful peacetime role – to wage agricultural war against the various pests and insects that damage crops. Shortly after came the realisation that other similarly structured, synthesised chemicals could be employed to great profit to 'improve' our way of life and consumer products. Coinciding with post-war prosperity, higher standards of living in the developed world and increased demand for luxuries as opposed to essentials, much of the chemical industry's innovation was focused on making life easier – and so the industry exploded with thousands of novel molecular structures. This from Du Pont in the fifties:

'Better things for better living....through chemistry'

....thereby heralding the coming of age of non-stick, easy-clean, disposable living. But, as most of us know from experience, just as there is no such thing as a free lunch, there's nearly always a downside when things come too easily – and this is one part of the story of man-made chemicals production at the turn of the 21st century. Synthetic chemicals are largely employed in consumer products to make things appear to be better, easier-to-use, longer-lasting, smoother-gliding and so on. But how keen would the average consumer be on a product if it also offered a significant dose of toxicity as part of that new-and-improved formula? There is a growing body of evidence which suggests that certain chemicals found in everyday products can compromise fertility and jeopardise the normal development of the foetus in utero. Furthermore, they may be disruptive to neurological function and the normal processes of the body's own chemical messaging system (the endocrine or hormone system) and are implicated in causing cancer. What is more, many chemicals build up in our body fat and never leave.

Arguably the last few decades have been a three-way conspiracy of ignorance between short-sighted, high-profit, quick-fix invention, keen consumer-driven desire for everything new-and-improved and extraordinary regulatory laxity. It's a situation that has resulted in some sectors of the chemicals industry single-handedly, and with great speed contaminating all four corners of the world. Toxic man-made chemicals are now an unavoidable global issue. They are found in places far removed from the factories that create them and the lifestyles that use the products containing them. They are in the air we breathe, the water we drink, the food we eat, the very earth under our feet – and they are in us: in our fat, blood, livers, brains and even in our new-born babies.

Chemical Dependency

The chemical industry is vast. It's responsible for about 7% of the world's GNP (Gross National Product) and employs over ten million people globally. It is important to state that we have a lot to thank this industry for. Many of the things we take for granted in modern life are due to the spectacular innovations of this sector such as precursors (a chemical compound that leads to another, usually more stable product) for pharmaceuticals, pigments for dyes and monomers to make plastics. However since the industry took off in the 1940's and 50's, the number of new chemical compounds that have been manufac-tured has been staggering. Well over 80 000 in the last fifty years with hundreds of new ones being added each year – and thousands of these have been released into the environment. More staggering is the number of these chemicals that are in the products that we use intimately in everyday life, the ones we slather over our skin, wrap our food in, paint on our finger nails, clean our cookers with, lay on our floors and put straight into the mouths of our babies. Most extraordinary of all is that the vast majority of these chemicals have never been adequately tested for their safety to the person or the environment. Of the ones that have been tested, few have been subjected to sufficient rigour. For example, a chemical might have been tested for its effect on a healthy, fully grown male, but not for how it may effect the foetus in utero.

> *"Given our understanding of the way chemicals interact with the environment, you could say we are running a gigantic experiment with humans and all other living things as the subject"*
> **Tom Blundell**
> **Chairman of UK Royal Commission on Environmental Pollution**

Post World War II, our average chance of getting cancer has risen from 1 in 4 to 1 in 3. While it would be impossible and totally misleading to lay all the blame at the feet of toxic chemicals, evidence is growing that they, along with several other lifestyle factors, have a significant influence on rising rates of cancer. The fact that, as consumers, our exposure to these chemicals is largely involuntary is something we ought to be increasingly concerned about.

Consenting Adults

Most of us do things from time to time that we know can have a negative impact on our health: drink alcohol, eat saturated fats or smoke cigarettes for example. Sometimes we do these things in moderation; sometimes we do them to excessive and dangerous levels. But whatever your vice and however much you indulge it, it is at least a choice made with an awareness of the risks attached. This book is concerned with toxic chemicals that have either proven or strongly implicated effects on our health, but which we are often exposed to without any choice. They are chemicals that we don't even know are there. There is a long list of everyday consumer products that we use frequently that contain an incredible number of synthetic chemicals, the effects of which on our health – short, medium and long term – are largely unknown. Current research has shown many synthetic chemicals to be toxic and implicated in a range of health issues including behavioural problems, declining sperm counts, neurological impairment, birth defects, allergies, diabetes and various cancers.

Furthermore, as well as being everywhere, many toxic chemicals also act promiscuously, leeching from the product that originally contained them and contaminating the wider environment. They can enter the food chain and are capable of travelling such vast distances on global airstreams that there is probably not a single species of living thing or a solitary area of this earth that remains uncontaminated by man-made chemicals. Think of the pristine vistas of the polar ice caps, visions of seemingly cool purity – incredibly these arctic regions are now polluted with some of the most toxic chemicals on the planet, as are the people and wildlife that live there.

So why are we so blissfully, if dangerously, ignorant? Largely because for many decades, the chemical industry could put products on the market with little or no safety testing and it was only when there was a problem that they were then removed. The onus of proof of danger was not with the industry producing the chemical – it was more a question of showing that damage was done. So now we have tens of thousands of inadequately tested chemicals in products and an ever-growing body of scientific evidence showing worrying health implications

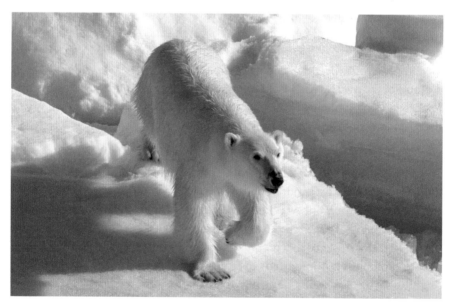

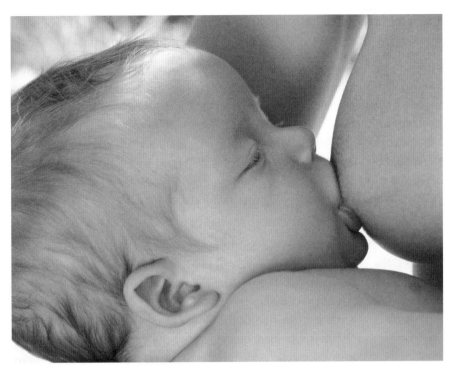

associated with a significant number of them. Since the harmful consequences of many common toxic chemicals do not become apparent for years, sometimes decades, by the time negative effects to health can be shown significant contamination has already occurred and irreversible harm done. For example, although a group of chemicals called PCBs are now banned, we will be living with their toxic legacy for hundreds of years. In the case of DDT, banned in this country in the seventies, all of us will probably have it in our blood – even if we were born yesterday.

This is because the effects of some of the most threatening chemicals can be long-term, building up in our body fat over years and being transferred both in the uterine environment, via breast milk, and through the food chain to our children. Others have more short-term influences, but if exposure happens at the wrong time, for example to a pregnant woman, the effects on her unborn child can be profound. It is important to realise that there are many products that ought really to carry warnings. 'Use this at your own risk – it contains chemicals that have not been properly tested for their short or medium, far less long-term effects on humans, wildlife or the environment and the most recent scientific evidence is giving us cause for concern.' So far they don't, so it really is up to us to find out for ourselves.

As long ago as 1962, an American biologist called Rachel Carson wrote a ground breaking book called 'Silent Spring', (in reference to the season rather than the water source). In it she warned of the dire potential fallout of the previous quarter century's contamination of life on earth by toxic, man-made chemicals:

'For the first time in the history of the world, every human being is now subjected to contact with dangerous chemicals, from the moment of their conception until death'

Close to half a century later, her major concerns relating to pesticides and insecticides have proven accurate and although many of these have now been strictly regulated or banned, they often still persist. Catastrophic levels of these older, potent chemicals were released recklessly into the environment in modern industrialised nations and given as aid to Africa. They are now still poisoning the breast milk of all women, but particularly Inuit women living in the Arctic. This will be explained in the last chapter which relates to the broader environmental consequences of chemicals. But at this stage, it's mentioned to highlight the incredible potency of some man-made chemicals.

Thankfully, due to improved science and the start of better regulation, contamination levels of those older chemicals, referred to by Rachel Carson, are finally dropping. But we still have to be mindful of the potential of other new chemicals that have a similar structure and thus might have similar effects. Equally, and perhaps even more worryingly, we need to understand how they might act together in so-called 'toxic cocktails'. Since 'Silent Spring' was published, tens of thousands more new chemicals have been produced with little or no testing for their potential impact on our health or environment. Fortunately, the tide is now turning and there is a growing awareness of the serious issues relating to many synthetic chemicals. However, since many of the newer chemicals are not as persistent or bioaccumulative, we might see worrying health effects yet not be able to identify which chemical is responsible because it has already broken down and left the body. Environmental groups such as WWF, Friends of the Earth and Greenpeace have worked very hard and been successful in getting these issues taken seriously at top governmental and regulatory body levels, despite intense dissembling and resistance from certain sectors of the chemical industry. One major reason for the environmental groups' success is that it is now impossible to ignore the results of important research and the irrefutable, observable effects of certain synthetic chemicals over time. The time for tighter control and rigour is now and most developed countries are putting the subject of toxic chemicals – significant environmental pollutants – high up the political agenda, not only nationally but internationally as well.

It is not the intention of this book to criticise the entire chemical industry. It is an industry that has immeasurably improved modern life, but like all powerful industries it needs to be adequately regulated. This is not yet the case. It is essential that the general public is aware of the inherent dangers of certain common chemicals and knows where they are to be found. We are not pretending to have all the answers, much more research needs to be completed before definitive facts are widely available for public information purposes. What we are saying is that in the case of synthetic chemicals with suspected toxicity, where we really don't know the full extent of their potential effects, we should err on the side of caution. There are enough examples of serious negative impacts on our health in recent times to make this the only sensible solution. Understanding some straightforward facts about synthetic chemicals, their widespread use in contemporary manufacturing – and how the toxicity of some can affect health and well-being will assist individuals in making informed choices about what products they choose to buy and use in the home, on holiday, in the car, in the office or schoolroom. This book will help its readers to become more aware of the extent to which we are all exposed to dangerous chemicals and offer alternatives to help minimise exposure, thereby improving health and longevity. Since it is no longer possible to totally avoid harmful chemicals, taking measures to reduce exposure is the only sensible option for individuals, governments and industry alike. Furthermore, consumer knowledge and its collective influence on purchasing can contribute to demanding that industry provides us with cleaner, greener and non-toxic options.

1

What are toxic chemicals and how do we get exposed to them?

In this book we will present the framework required to understand the hazardous role that everyday toxic chemicals play in contemporary lifestyles. We will detail the most worrying substances and where to find them, describe the main ways that we are exposed to them and explain what it is about certain chemicals that makes them such a cause for concern, personally and environmentally. We will show that although toxic chemicals are an unavoidable fact of life, simply by knowing what and where they are you can take action to reduce your exposure significantly, thereby improving the quality of your immediate environment and protecting you and your family's health.

What is toxic? – In a broad sense an easier question to ask would be what's not toxic? Even water, if too much of it is consumed at once, can be harmful and even potentially fatal. A toxic substance, however, generally relates to any substance that enters the environment in a quantity or concentration that may have an immediate or long-term effect on that environment or on human or animal life and health. A **toxin**, on the other hand, relates to poisonous substances produced in nature, by certain plants, animals or bacteria that can harm or kill other living organisms – like snake venom, a bee sting or botulism. We are not dealing with toxins here.

A **toxic chemical**, for the purposes of this book, is a man-made (synthetic) chemical, primarily produced out of organic (ie. carbon-based) chemistry, which is released into the environment in concentrations sufficient to have the potential to cause harm to humans, animals or the environment. In some cases, those levels are almost too small to imagine, particularly when considering the effects on the foetus developing in utero. Naturally occurring toxic chemicals such as lead and cadmium also exist and can present serious health risks, but we will only be covering man-made chemicals.

Determining the toxicity of a chemical can be very difficult. The concentration and length of exposure required to cause harmful effects can vary widely. Assessing the toxicity of all the possible variations of chemicals working together to create a **cocktail effect** is virtually impossible. It may be the case that an individual chemical is shown to be 'safe', but when exposure is in combination with another, or others, toxic effects may occur. The reality is that we are never exposed to one chemical at a time, in everyday life we are exposed to a huge chemical cocktail. Additive effects are being seen in laboratory experiments and it is likely that there will be similar effects in humans too. Hence the authors of this book advocate a policy of caution and minimisation of exposure to chemicals where toxicity has been shown to be harmful or potentially so. We believe this is the only sensible course of action for governments and industry as well (see Chapter 5).

We are primarily concerned with **synthetic chemicals** used in the manufacture of common consumer products: from nail polish to cars. We are not dealing with agrochemicals ie. agricultural pesticides and insecticides. Where we do touch on food it is in relation to the way it is packaged, processed and prepared.

Our baseline advice with respect to what you eat is as follows;

- Ensure that as much of your diet as possible comes from as low down the food chain as possible ie. plenty of fresh fruit and vegetables
- Choose organic produce if available
- Avoid processed food
- Ensure that any meat or fish consumption is from known, 'clean' sources (eg. The Atlantic is less polluted than the Mediterranean so it's generally better to buy fish from the former than the latter) and again, organic wherever possible.

Be aware that the food we eat is generally subject to the phenomena of bioaccumulation and biomagnification detailed below. Even organic meat and fish, by being higher up the food chain than vegetables for example, will contain significant concentrations of common toxic chemicals. We are not advocating vegetarianism, just moderation, balance and a generally healthy eating regime.

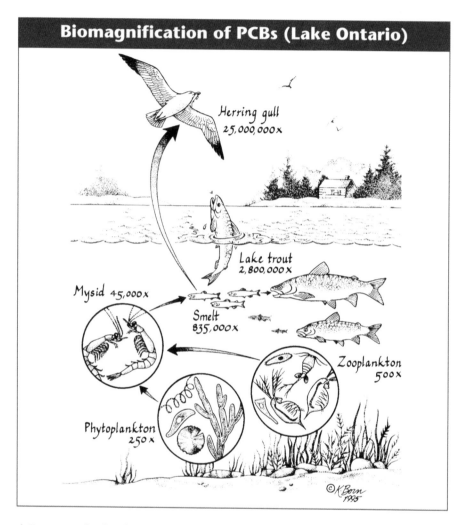

Biomagnification of PCBs (Lake Ontario)

Herring gull
25,000,000x

Lake trout
2,800,000x

Mysid 45,000x

Smelt
835,000x

Zooplankton
500x

Phytoplankton
250x

©K Born
1995

'Organic' chemicals?

Not to be confused with organic foods and products, organic chemicals are simply compounds of hydrogen and carbon synthesised artificially in places like the laboratory. Organic chemistry is the foundation from which modern, man-made chemicals are produced and has given rise to a whole array of plastics, solvents, flame retardants, preservatives, water-proofers, plasticisers, surfactants and many other substances used in the production of consumer goods.

22

Key features of toxic chemicals

Persistent chemicals are those that don't readily break down in the environment, but linger for years, sometimes decades. When chemicals don't break down and are continually released into the environment, their concentration will inevitably increase. If a persistent chemical is also toxic then widespread and worrying contamination can occur (see Chapter 2 on PCBs).

Fat-Loving Molecules – many chemicals are predominantly **lipophilic** in nature, which literally means lipid-loving or fat-loving so they don't readily dissolve in water – this makes them hard to metabolise. Once they've entered the body they tend to remain in the fatty tissues, including the fat content of the blood, brain and liver etc. If a substance is both lipophilic and persists in the environment, then it can be readily taken up by organisms from contaminated environments such as soil and water. From there it can **bioaccumulate** in the food chain and then every time something higher up the food chain eats something contaminated below it, the concentration increases exponentially by a process called **biomagnification.** By the time it reaches the top of the food chain, the concentration of a persistent, bioaccumulative chemical can be many **millions** of times that of the original environmental contamination. Persistence, toxicity and bioaccumulation results in a **toxic body burden**, which may lead to a toxic effect.

PBT Chemicals – a term used to describe the above traits when present in the same chemical, ie. persistent, bioaccumulative & toxic.

Persistent Organic Pollutants (POPs) are chemicals that exhibit, to a dangerous degree, the three criteria of PBTs: persistence, toxicity and bioaccumulation. POPs are known to be extremely hazardous and examples include pesticides (eg. DDT), industrial chemicals (eg. PCB) and the by-products of industrial processes (eg. Dioxins and Furans). These chemicals now surround us in daily life and we are constantly exposed to them. POPs are capable of travelling through water and air to regions far away from their source and can span boundaries of geography and generations. The twelve most potent and most dangerous to human (and wildlife) health are known as the dirty dozen and are already strictly regulated under a United Nations global treaty known as The Stockholm Convention (2001), commonly called the POPs Convention. Several organisations like WWF feel that many more chemicals with similar characteristics should be added to the list. For example, certain BFRs (brominated flame retardants – see Chapter 2) – a chemical group widely used to prevent common consumer products from going up in flames too quickly in the event of fire. Although flame retardants undoubtedly save lives, some safer alternatives with less toxic side effects are available and more need to be developed for widespread application.

Endocrine-Disrupting Chemicals (EDCs) are chemicals that can interfere with the endocrine or hormone system – the body's own chemical messaging system. Our hormones regulate bodily functions such as metabolism, sexual development and growth. Hormones are released into the blood by various glands including the testicles, ovaries and thyroid and include the sex hormones oestrogen (female) and testosterone (male). The endocrine system is a finely balanced one, and profoundly connected to the nervous and immune systems. Since the most minuscule levels of hormone have great effect, endocrine-disrupting chemicals can play havoc with nature – particularly at crucial stages of development and especially during the complex process of development before birth (see Chapter 3). EDCs have a variety of end-points; they can block natural hormone action, mimic it or have an opposing effect. Chemicals that interfere with the sex hormones in this way are commonly referred to in the popular media as 'gender-benders'. EDC effects were first seen in wildlife and while much subsequent research has been done on animal subjects, similar effects are becoming increasingly evident in humans. Various experiments have shown that EDCs found in common consumer products are implicated in both sexual malformations and confused sexual behaviour in animals. There is a growing body of scientific research findings that suggests a link between certain EDCs and reproductive system birth defects, sperm count decline and sexually related cancers in humans. (1 - see references on page 126)

Leaching – the problem with some chemicals is that they do not stay locked inside products they are originally added to and can **leach** out during normal everyday use of that product. They can accumulate in house dust, in the air, in food and can contribute to indoor pollution as well as contaminating the more general environment. A chemical that leaches out of a product can be called a

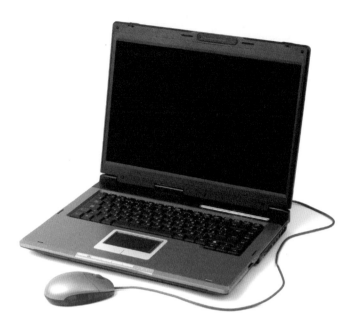

leachate. Common examples are bisphenol A, a chemical used to line food cans and which can leach into the contents, or certain flame retardants that leach out of the plastic casings of electrical equipment like TV's or computers and into the air.

VOCs – Volatile Organic Compounds – these are compounds which have the ability to evaporate or readily vaporise at room temperature. If these compounds are toxic, then they will contribute to indoor air pollution and potentially pose a risk to health and well-being. Paints, cleaning products, glues, PVC flooring, MDF/particle board, carpeting and polishes all commonly contain VOCs and may 'off-gas' into the environment around them. **Formaldehyde is one of the most common VOCs in domestic environments** (see Chapter 2).

Off-gassing is the process whereby gaseous pollutants release from the objects and products they are in, into the environment. This generally applies to VOCs found in paint, certain plastics, cleaning products, PVC flooring, carpet backing, particle board and so on.

25

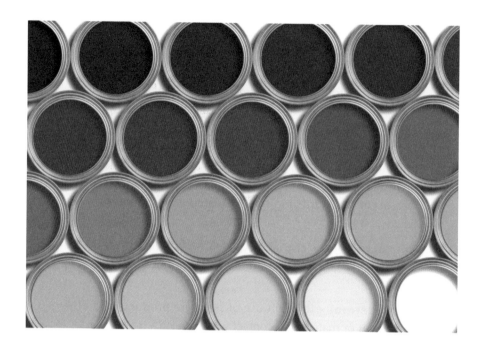

The toxic body burden

The term **toxic body burden** refers to the amount of toxic chemicals that are present in the body at any given time. We are constantly exposed to chemicals, both naturally occurring substances and synthetic ones, to those that are toxic and those that are not. Whether and how a chemical enters the body, and how long it stays there, depends on the intrinsic nature of the substance and the degree of exposure. Exposure can vary according to the state the chemical is in (liquid, gaseous, solid etc.), the prevailing environmental conditions and, in the case of consumer products, according to how we use the products that contain it. Some chemicals are readily metabolised (broken down and excreted) by the body. Others, that are persistent and bioaccumulative, can remain in our tissues for decades. Even in the case of easily metabolised chemicals, if exposure to them is daily then they will be a constant factor in our overall toxic body burden. Though the level may vary, everyone has a toxic body burden whether they live in a city high-rise or an isolated smallholding in the countryside, by the seaside or next to an industrial plant.

Main exposure routes:

- **Ingestion** – from eating foods that have been contaminated with toxic chemicals: this may be through bioaccumulation in the food chain, from food production processes or from its subsequent packaging. However they get there, fatty foods are more likely to be harbouring bioaccumulative or lipophilic toxic chemicals than non-fatty foods (although toxicity from agrochemicals also affects many if not most non-organic fruit and vegetables). Exposure can also occur from drinking contaminated water, milk and other liquids.

- **Inhalation** – toxic chemicals can leach out of the products that contain them into the air, creating both indoor and outdoor pollution.

- **Trans-dermal** – through use of skin care products and other substances or materials in contact with our skin.

- **Through the placenta and breast milk** – the foetus will necessarily receive some of its mother's toxic body burden through the placenta and, after birth, the baby will receive more through breast milk. This is an unavoidable reality of living in such chemical times. It is generally accepted that a mother will pass on approximately 30% of her own toxic body burden to her first-born child. The authors of this book do not advise against breast feeding – it is the best possible start for a baby, providing the perfect balance of nutrients and immunity, and it is vital for mother and baby bonding. What we do believe is that breast milk and the womb should not be contaminated by synthetic toxic chemicals in the first place, and so we encourage minimising your exposure to them.

- **Intravenous** – a stay in hospital can expose the individual to toxic chemicals such as phthalates (see Chapter 2) which can leach out of the soft plastic blood bags and medical tubing into the liquids (eg. drugs or blood) they contain and then into the patient.

How do we know what our toxic body burden is?

The short answer is that we don't unless we have ourselves **biomonitored** and even then only a limited picture will emerge. Biomonitoring is a process whereby analyses are performed on samples of blood, adipose (fatty) tissue, breast milk, urine etc to assess whether certain substances are present and in what concentrations. It is virtually impossible for these tests to be exhaustive because the number of chemicals that could be looked at is enormous and the process is expensive. What tends to happen is that a list of chemicals is defined at the start of the biomonitoring testing and the samples provided are tested for levels of those chemicals. These lists can be long and provide fascinating insights into the spectrum of contamination.

Knowing the extent of one's personal body burden may encourage the individual to try to actively minimise their exposure to known and suspected toxic chemicals. However, where biomonitoring is most useful is in organised testing of the population as a whole to track 'toxic trends' and to act as an early warning system for the newer toxic chemicals entering the environment and the food chain. Various NGOs (non-government organisations), notably WWF and governments, such as the Swedish, have conducted 'snapshot' biomonitoring programmes that have given a contamination overview – in some cases comparing regional, lifestyle and generational factors. Though some studies have not been extensive enough to be representative of the population at large, these studies have provided some interesting insights:

- We are all contaminated, even in the womb – a location we idealistically associate with safety and the best possible environment for the nurturing of a developing child. A joint WWF UK/Greenpeace investigation into hazardous chemicals in umbilical cords tested those of over 30 newborn babies for 35 synthetic chemicals. The results revealed that between 5 and 14 of the chemicals tested for were in their bodies already. Most of those chemicals are found in normal everyday products in the home (see Chapter 6)

- In terms of our toxic body burdens, there does not appear to be a significant advantage to living in the country rather than the city. There is a prevailing

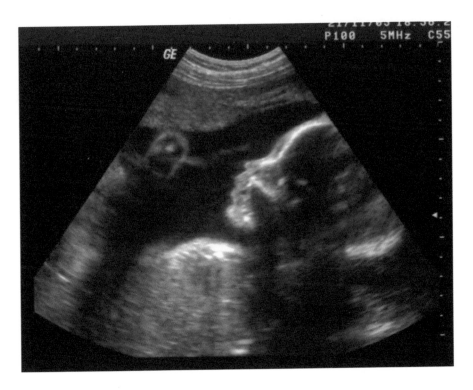

assumption that rural living is healthier and cleaner. Unfortunately, in terms of toxic man-made chemical contamination, this does not appear to be the case. What you eat may be more of a factor than where you live (see below) as may be your indoor environments: your home, car and workplace too

- The overwhelming majority of people tested by the WWF biomonitoring programme had toxic chemicals found in everyday household products in their blood. It is impossible to say how they got there, but hard to avoid the implication that if people are living in intimate contact with these products and the chemicals are able to leach out of the products into the domestic environment, then it is likely that this is a key exposure route

- PCBs, which are found in elevated levels in oily fish, have been found to be at higher concentrations in the blood of individuals whose lifestyle question-naires revealed that they ate more oily fish than other people tested in the same sample

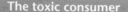

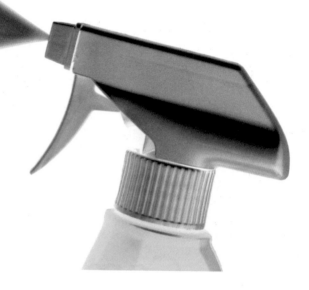

- The WWF cross-generational biomonitoring survey of 2004 tested and compared toxic body burdens of three generations of the same families. The results showed that, despite having had less time to accrue a body burden, children were sometimes contaminated with higher concentrations than their parents and grandparents. While the older generations tended to have more of the 'older' chemicals in their blood (DDT, PCBs etc) the children showed elevated levels of more 'modern' toxic chemicals like brominated flame retardants (BFRs – used extensively in soft furnishings, electrical equipment and textiles) and perfluorinates (common in non-stick pans, water-resistant clothing and footwear)

It is becoming increasingly apparent that, despite the myriad of lifestyle factors that affect our general health and well-being, when it comes to toxic chemicals what we know for certain is that we don't yet know how dangerous they are. However, there is sufficient evidence to warrant serious cause for concern and until we know for certain, products that contain toxic chemicals need to be taken off the market or their toxic elements be replaced with safer alternatives. Meanwhile, the fact that these chemicals are not commonly signposted as being dangerous on labelling means that we need to be as aware as possible in order to minimise our exposure. The next chapter introduces the most common toxic chemicals found in consumer products.

2

Common toxic
chemicals:
Ten to watch

The following introduction to ten of the most common toxic chemicals found in consumer products is not intended to scare or induce sudden paranoia – we have to accept that they are frequently, if not always, there – but rather to inform, so that exposure to them can be reduced to safer levels and consumers can start to choose and demand safer, cleaner, greener options. Some toxic chemicals have been well studied and their toxic effects clearly documented. Others, much more worryingly, are added to our consumer products despite very little testing, making us all guinea pigs. Since the reason for the creation of many of the following chemicals is often to provide resistance and resilience in consumer goods – making them water-proof, non-stick, flame resistant and to act as preservatives – it is perhaps not a huge surprise that they have become such pervasive global contaminants. Some of the following compounds are persistent, bioaccumulative and toxic (PBTs), some are endocrine disruptors and some others are so ubiquitous that our day-to-day exposure to them is pretty constant. Of course, amongst the tens of thousands of synthesised chemicals in widespread use many more than ten show worrying profiles and we will also be making passing references to other less studied compounds during the course of this book. It may well be that the vast majority of synthetic chemicals are 'safe', but at the moment all we know for certain is that we don't know.

PCB – an example of how it can, and did, go horribly wrong

PCB stands for polychlorinated biphenyl. There are over 200 variants. PCBs are classic PBTs (ie, persistent, bioaccumulative and toxic). First synthesised in the late 1800's, PCBs went into commercial production in the 1920's. They were swiftly adopted by the electrical industry when they proved to be super-effective insulators and coolants in electrical equipment due to their robust and non-flammable qualities. PCBs also found their way into the home in a whole host of consumer products such as flame retardants and rubber preservatives and were used as additives in paints, varnishes, printing inks, some pesticides, strip lights and carbonless copy paper. As early as the 1930's, there were reports of toxic effects in people working in PCB manufacturing plants: some of whom were developing an unsightly pustular skin condition called Chloracne and complaining of other negative health effects. It wasn't until the mid-sixties that the wider consequences of PCBs began to become apparent. Almost by chance a Swedish scientist, Dr Soren Jensen, who was investigating blood levels of another toxic chemical, DDT, discovered that not only were PCBs ubiquitous in terms of their use in manufactured products, but they were everywhere else too: rampant in the Swedish environment, in the soil, water and animals. Further tests revealed them to be in himself, his wife and his young children as well. On the publication of his findings the global scientific community began to investigate and it became apparent that PCBs were disrupting food webs and contaminating environments all over the planet.

During this time it is unclear whether major producers and users of PCBs (companies such as Monsanto and General Electric) were aware of the extent of the toxic nature of the product that they were selling and discharging huge quantities of into the environment. It took over a decade, much litigation and a huge body of research worldwide before Monsanto was finally prevented from manufacturing these hazardous toxic chemicals (except for use in 'totally enclosed' systems). Litigation continues to this day with respect to responsibility for various clean-up operations relating to PCB contamination of the Hudson River in the United States, but the full fallout of PCB contamination will never be fully quantifiable. There have been reports of young men rendered infertile due to their exposure, legions of skin disorders, PCB workers dying of skin cancer, dolphins carrying over seventeen times the concentration of PCBs in their blubber required to classify them as toxic waste, related birth defects and developmental problems in exposed children. The Arctic has effectively become a dumping ground for PCBs and other persistent organic pollutants (POPs), the majority of which are organochlorine compounds released by industries in developed regions like the US and Europe which lie at the lower latitudes. The compounds are swept into the Arctic by prevailing winds, diffusing quickly and easily into the atmosphere. Inuit women from the Arctic regions, thousands of miles from any industrial source, have become so contaminated that many have to think twice about breast-feeding their babies because of the PCB concentration in their breast milk.

Other studies on the health effects associated with exposure to PCBs indicated neuro-toxicity (harmful to the nervous system including the brain), reproductive and developmental toxicity, immune system suppression, liver damage, skin irritation, endocrine disruption and probable carcinogenicity.

PCBs are classic 'legacy' chemicals, so called because they will be contaminating the environment and living things for generations. They are so widely dispersed that they show up in the wombs of pregnant women and in whales in the deepest oceans and yet there is no known way to get rid of them apart from the passing of hundreds of years and the slow amelioration of their potent toxic effect. (A recent biomonitoring survey by WWF found that PCB levels in the blood were significantly lower than a decade ago proving that strict regulation does work when properly enforced.) The story of PCBs is like the fictional invention of a horror-story writer and demonstrates,

a) that a chemical should not be put on the market prior to full testing to ensure it is 'safe' – and that this should be the responsibility of the chemical company manufacturing the chemical

b) the importance of strong regulation to prevent companies from ducking their responsibilities with loop-holes and 'get out' clauses. If a chemical is shown to be a PBT (persistent, bioaccumulative and toxic), it should never go on the market to be used in consumer goods. Even after the case of PCBs – classic PBTs – the lessons don't seem to have been learnt. Chemicals with similar properties to the PCBs such as some BFRs – brominated flame retardants, (see page 35) and perfluorinates (see page 39) are still in widespread use in everyday products. We need to learn lessons from the recent past.

TEN TO WATCH OUT FOR AND AVOID WHERE POSSIBLE:

1. BROMINATED FLAME RETARDANTS (BFRs)

What are they and what threat do they pose?

Brominated flame retardants are synthetic chemicals that are added to many consumer goods including furnishings, carpeting, bedding, children's clothing and electrical goods so that, in the event of a fire, they will burn more slowly. BFRs can be persistent, bioaccumulative and toxic and have endocrine-disrupting properties – particularly thyroid imbalances. [2 - see references on page 126]

Negative health effects have been shown on the liver, the brain and the nervous system when tested on animals. Recently there has been a sharp rise recorded in levels of BFRs in human breast milk. When such chemicals are impregnated into products like mattresses and sofas, items we have close, long-lasting and regular contact with, this is extremely worrying. Where BFRs are shown to be PBT then humans, wildlife and the environment should be protected from exposure to them and their use should be banned where exposure can occur. There is more and more evidence that the levels of concentration of some of these persistent, bioaccumulative and toxic chemicals in the environment, wildlife and our bodies is on the increase.

So are we becoming more flame retardant in the process? This is not necessarily a joke! Plenty of anecdotal evidence from those involved in the crematorium side of the funeral business suggests that, for one reason or another, the modern corpse takes longer to burn and at a hotter temperature than our ancestors did. While we're on the subject, those choosing the burial option may find themselves taking longer to decompose too (this is possibly due to elevated levels of various chemical 'preservatives' in our bodies). Whatever the truth of the effects in the hereafter, in the here and now brominated flame retardants are posing quite a problem for the environment, wildlife and human health. In contrast to the flames they are designed to suppress, BFRs have spread like wildfire in the environment and are now a major global contaminant.

It should be pointed out that there is a legal requirement for certain consumer goods to be treated with flame retardants, although ironically one of the major reasons for this is because an increasing number of consumer goods are being manufactured from synthetic materials which tend to burn faster than natural ones. (You may remember that when the first plastic TV and computer casings began to appear, they had a tendency to catch fire from the heat generated by components inside – this was when cheap and available bromines began to be employed to make flame retardants and their use started to become widespread). Commonly, it is the polyurethane foam in soft furnishings, the plastic casing of small electrical goods like computers and televisions and carpeting and floorings with synthetic fibres that contain the highest BFR content (up to 10% of the products overall content in some cases). Many natural fibres, especially when tightly woven, and other natural materials do not require treatment with flame-retardants, or if they do it is to a much lesser degree. The presence of BFRs in consumer products has undoubtedly saved lives and obviously we do not want people to burn in their beds, but the wholesale infusion of numerous common products with a proven global contaminant is a far from ideal solution to the risk of fire. Safer, less toxic alternatives need to be developed for general use.

Facts about retardants

- The most common, most studied and most worrying brominated flame retardants are the PBDEs (poly-brominated diphenyl ethers). There are three main variants, Penta-BDE, Octa-BDE and Deca-BDE and over 200 individual chemicals in the 'family'

- The EU has banned Penta–BDE and Octa-BDE. The third common variant, Deca-BDE, is still in use but under constant scrutiny because there is the distinct possibility that it 'de-brominates' into the more worrying forms that are being phased out and Deca itself is suspected of posing health risks

- BFRs, particularly certain PBDEs, can rapidly build up in the environment and in living things, including humans. They are now embedded in the global food web and are showing up in ever-increasing concentrations in the blubber of whales from remote and deep Atlantic waters and in the breast milk of women all over the world. Because of this, certain PBDEs have been put forward by various NGOs, agencies and governments for inclusion within the POPs convention (see Chapter 6)

- Chemically, PBDEs are very similar to PCBs and both have structural similarities to thyroid hormone. PBDEs have effects on thyroid and hormone balance and are reported to have neurotoxic effects. [3 - ref. see page 126] Of special concern is exposure to PBDEs in utero since they can be taken up during neonatal life, concentrate in the brain and may have neurotoxic effects at crucial stages of development

- In some countries, the concentrations of PBDEs in human breast milk have been doubling every five years. Sweden took swift and early action, banning PBDEs in the 1990's, and levels are now declining

- The EU ecolabel already excludes brominated flame retardants, and Dell has said it intends to apply. Both NEC and Phillips are working to replace brominated flame retardants.

What products are they in and how do they get into me?

- Sofas and other soft furnishings, carpets and rugs (especially those with synthetic fibre content), electrical goods (such as the housing for computers, TVs, DVD players, mobile phones, MP3 players, laptops, PDAs), car interiors, public transport interiors, offices, various textiles and some clothing brands (they can even be found in some school uniforms and kids' pyjamas)

- There are two main exposure routes, firstly through the food chain and secondly via inhalation as BFRs are widely found in the dust that collects on household floors and on objects such as computer keyboards. They release from the objects that originally contain them and contaminate the indoor, as well as outdoor, environment. They can also be passed on to the foetus through the placenta and to the baby via breast milk.

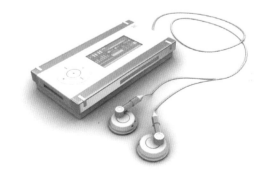

Alternatives

- Many companies, partly in anticipation of a possible ban on all PBDEs, are working to replace BFRs with greener, cleaner alternatives. Dell, Ericsson, Philips, IKEA and NEC are all actively seeking and using less toxic solutions

- IKEA has phased out all BFRs from their products

- Minimise the goods in your home that are treated with PBDEs and when buying new goods check for less toxic or toxic-free alternatives. Choose tightly woven natural fabrics for your domestic textile requirements (curtains, furniture covers, bed linen and so on) and opt for wooden or plant-based flooring (like sisal or coir matting) instead of carpeting. Choose computers and other electrical goods with metal as opposed to plastic casings

- Keep house dust to a minimum and keep all rooms well-ventilated

- To minimise exposure to BFRs you could furnish your home with older, pre-BFR furniture such as antiques and actively pursue a preventative approach to the domestic fire risk (though this must be your free, calculated risk – furthermore in some rented accommodation, it is a legal requirement that the furnishings comply with fire regulations if manufactured after the date that the regulations came into force). Generally, unplug electrical appliances when not in use (don't leave them on stand-by), install proper fire alarms, don't smoke in bed and don't deep fat fry at home – you know it's not good for you anyway!

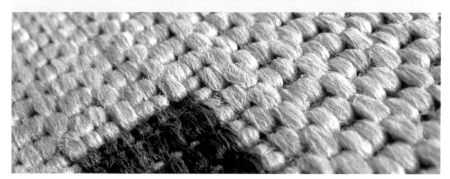

2. PERFLUORINATES OR PFCs

What are they and what threat do they pose?

Perfluorinates such as PFOS (Perfluorooctane sulfonate) and PFOA (Perfluorooctanoic acid) are the group of chemicals that make it easy to fry eggs without them sticking to the pan, that keep the rain off our backs when we face the elements and protect our carpets, shoes and furniture from getting stained. These chemicals have strong water and oil-repelling properties, a near imperviousness to heat and are to be found in a number of well-known consumer brands of non-stick, non-stain or water-resistant products. They are probably one of the most widespread toxic chemicals and are found in us, and other living things all over the globe, in levels that are increasingly a cause for concern. Because they do not degrade and are very persistent, they are sometimes referred to as 'eternal' compounds. Exposure to perfluorinated chemicals such as PFOS and PFOA may cause birth defects, adversely affect the immune system and disrupt thyroid function. (4 - see references on page 126). If exposure happens during pregnancy other developmental problems may ensue. The expanding knowledge about fluorochemicals in the environment again raises the question of how they could spread so widely before being comprehensively studied by regulatory bodies. This is a classic case of industry not taking responsibility for its chemicals and not adequately testing them before putting them on the market. If you have a canary in your kitchen, beware! Teflon Toxicosis is a recognised and not uncommon cause of death amongst small house birds. Even when used at 'recommended' temperatures, non-stick cookware can give off toxic fumes that are potentially lethal to small birds. They die because the fumes cause their lungs to haemorrhage and fill with fluid resulting in their suffocation. There is also something known as polymer fume fever in humans which, although quite rare in the home, can happen if a non-stick pan is left on the heat and the temperature rises to over 662°F/350°C (some studies cite lower temperatures). At this point, the coating starts to break down into particulates and gases and they can easily be inhaled, or ingested with the food cooked on the non-stick coating.

Perfluorinate Facts

- PFOS was voluntarily phased out of use in Scotchguard products by producer 3M in 2001 because of evidence of the chemical's toxicity. However, PFOA is still currently used in other consumer products and is in widespread use

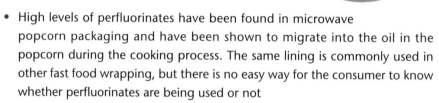

- It has been shown that some fish can break down other less toxic fluorinated chemicals into both PFOS and PFOA which then persist and bioaccumulate in the environment

- High levels of perfluorinates have been found in microwave popcorn packaging and have been shown to migrate into the oil in the popcorn during the cooking process. The same lining is commonly used in other fast food wrapping, but there is no easy way for the consumer to know whether perfluorinates are being used or not

- The US Environmental Protection Agency considers both PFOS and PFOA to be carcinogenic and occupational exposure to PFOS has been linked with increased occurrence of bladder cancer. They have recently come to an agreement with eight US manufacturers to change their manufacturing processes so as to reduce emissions of PFOA by 95% by 2010 and eliminate trace amounts of the compound in consumer products by 2015

- There are concerns over the concentration of perfluorinates in some children being as high as in adults despite having had far less time to be exposed to them. This may partly be due to the fact that they play on carpets and floors, more frequently wear clothes impregnated with perfluorinated chemicals and may be more sensitive to them

There are serious concerns about the use of PFOS in fire-fighting foam, so-called 'firewater', especially during big fires where it inevitably contaminates the surrounding environment and water supply and may contaminate vast areas and many thousands of people. (cf. The Buncefield disaster, Hertfordshire, UK, 2005 – a massive fire at an oil depot left over 12 million litres of highly toxic 'firewater' which has proved very tricky to dispose of without contaminating the local environment.)

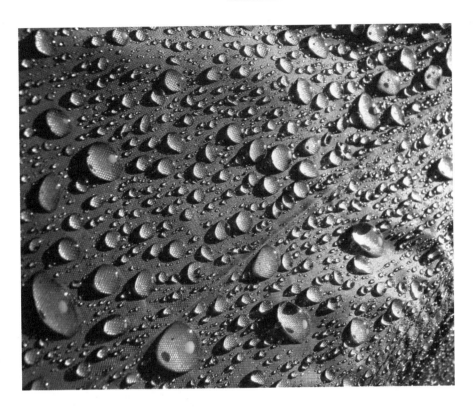

What products are they in and how do they get into me?

- Waterproof outdoor clothing (such as hiking boots, synthetic 'breathable' fabrics, ski wear etc.) crease resistant clothing (like school uniforms), carpets, upholstery, leather goods, floor waxes, non-stick cookware, occasionally inside ovens, in aerosol cans used to spray stain protector on to shoes and leather goods. They are also widely used on the inside of fast food containers to stop the grease from the food going through the wrapping

- The main exposure routes are thought to be ingestion via the contaminated food chain, through the inhalation of fumes and via the general degradation of products containing them, in the home environment, into house dust and air pollution

- Perfluorinates can also be passed on through the placenta and breast milk routes.

41

Alternatives

- In the kitchen choose stainless steel (the professional cook's choice), cast iron, ceramic titanium or porcelain enamelled cast iron

- If you do cook with non-stick cookware it's best to use it at temperatures as low as possible. Keep the kitchen well-ventilated and, to be on the safe side, ensure small birds, babies and children are well out of the way!

- Check the labels on your children's school uniforms for chemicals like Teflon and choose natural alternatives wherever possible. If school regulations insist on certain suppliers complain to the head teacher

- Avoid 'no ironing required' ranges of clothing

- Avoid fast food packaging, especially if it contains food with a high fat content – which is the vast majority of it

- If offered stain repellents when buying new furniture say no thank you.

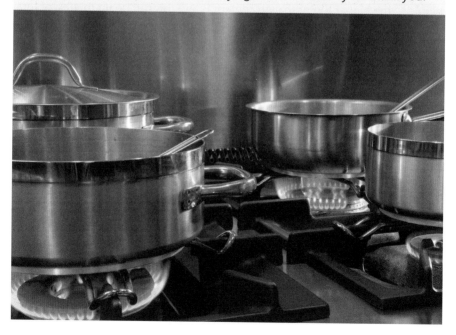

3. PHTHALATES – A FLEXIBLE FRIEND?

What are they and what threat do they pose?

A strange-looking word, but a very common chemical. Phthalates (the ph is silent when you say it) are produced in high volumes in manufacturing to make plastic products more flexible or less brittle and to give cosmetics that 'super-smooth' feel. Not all phthalates are a health concern, but the ones that are, are of great concern as they are endocrine disruptors, implicated in a range of 'feminising' effects and they are the classic 'leaching' chemical since they do not bind strongly with the original product they are added to. The most common form, and generally considered the most toxic, is DEHP (Di (2-ethylhexyl)pthalate). It's found in an extremely wide range of objects and places including some children's toys, car interiors, PVC (polyvinyl chloride) flooring (and fetish wear etc...!), blood bags, vinyl upholstery, shower curtains, plastic packaging, bags, all manner of moulded plastic objects and the ubiquitous credit card or charge card (The Co-operative Bank in association with WWF UK do offer a phthalate-free alternative). Generally, the more soft and flexible a phthalate-containing plastic is, the higher the phthalate content is and this can be up to 40% of total volume. This is incredible when you consider that a drum of industrial phthalate would carry a major health hazard warning and yet up until comparatively recently, a child's teething ring could be one third composed of it. In the EU, phthalates are now banned in toys and other products for the under three's and there are plans to ban more phthalate compounds in other children's toys and cosmetics.

However the effectiveness of this ban is questionable; it is suspected that many toys imported into the EU from places like the Far East are not checked and may contain the banned phthalates. A secondary, but equally common use of phthalates is as an additive in a vast range of cosmetics, personal care products, pharmaceuticals, paints, printing inks, sealants and adhesives – where their plasticiser properties are used to perform functions such as preventing nail varnish from chipping and make moisturisers slide more easily over skin. As flexible and prevalent as they are, phthalates are also very flexible contaminants, found universally in the environment, human body tissues and fluids such as breast milk and semen. Despite not being particularly persistent in the environment, their

commonplace usage means that they get topped up all the time and are a regular toxic guest in our bodies, often from multiple sources. Some phthalates are known endocrine disruptors and there is an increasing body of research showing they may be implicated in a range of health issues, perhaps most worryingly with regard to male reproductive development in utero, general increases in male reproductive impairment and the early onset of puberty and premature breast development in young girls.(5 - see references on page 126)
–(Also see Chapter 3)

Phthalate Facts

- Although individual products may contain relatively low concentrations of phthalates, when you sit down and add up all the different intimate exposures you might have in one day (especially if you use a full line-up of personal grooming products), it is easy to see how levels can build up. Especially since phthalates leach easily from products that contain them

- Phthalates have become one of the most abundant industrial pollutants in the world

- Products with phthalate content do not yet have to show that content on the label and often don't

- Despite only having a half life of around 12 hours, phthalates metabolites in the urine of women in one study (Hoppin et al 2002) are generally quite constant, suggesting a constant daily exposure

- A fascinating study into a high incidence of premature breast development in very young girls (8-24 months) in Puerto Rico concluded with the suggestion that high phthalate exposure during crucial stages of development could be responsible. One theory was that this was down to the high volume of plastic packaged food consumed there combined with the constant high temperatures and humidity.

What products are they in and how do they get into me?

- Flexible plastics, cosmetics, moulded plastic car dashboards, plastic food wrap, toothbrush handles, toys, shampoos

- In terms of how they get into us, the short answer is, in every way possible:

  - Ingestion: through biting and sucking objects with phthalate content and subsequent swallowing of the saliva (clearly this most commonly refers to babies and young children, but adult exceptions may also occur!)

  - Ingestion via food production and packaging

  - Inhalation from indoor air pollution, house dust

  - Transdermally from the legions of cosmetics and personal care products that contain phthalates

  - Through an intravenous drip, if you are receiving certain medical treatment from blood bags or from flexible medical tubing

  - From mother to child through the placenta and from breast milk.

Alternatives

- It's hard to avoid them, but increasingly manufacturers are advertising their plastics as being phthalate free, especially those aimed at babies and young children

- Choose personal grooming products that are free of any petrochemicals or synthetic additives

- Choose natural flooring over PVC

- Where there is an option, choose more rigid plastics over softer varieties

- Choose wooden or metal toys for your children.

4. BISPHENOL A or BPA or polycarbonate

What is it and what threat does it pose?

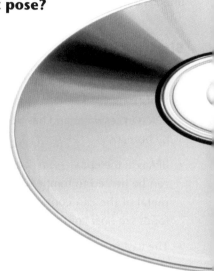

Although first synthesised as a synthetic oestrogen (a man-made hormone), bisphenol A was quickly adopted by the chemical industry when they discovered they could 'polymerise' it into polycarbonate, a plastic with many attractive properties such as low weight, high heat and electrical resistance, shatter resistance and optical clarity to boot. Endless uses beckoned, many of them within the food and drink packaging industry. Possibly it's only downside was that it was still effectively a synthetic oestrogen and that the bonds locking it together in the plastic could easily break, making it potentially quite a leaky sort of chemical to have come into intimate contact with food. This glaring disadvantage has not seemed to have affected bisphenol A's progress into relative indispensability. It's very big business with almost three million tonnes being produced annually in the world and, like the phthalates, it's very hard to avoid. It's in thousands of products. From baby feeding bottles to mobile phones, DVDs to plastic lunch boxes and spectacle lenses to the linings of baked bean cans – as well as in various floorings, composite building materials, paints, adhesives and dental sealants. And of course, because of its leaky nature, it is in us too.

If bisphenol A had ever been licensed as a pharmaceutical product, it would have gone through various tests and had clear dosage levels attached to it. It didn't because it was superseded by a more potent synthetic oestrogen called DES (a drug that itself had disastrous consequences for many pregnant women and their children in the '50's, '60's and early '70's – see Chapter 3). But as events turned out, we are all now getting varying and inadequately regulated doses of bisphenol A due to its widespread use in consumer products and the ability it has to leach from them into our food and drink, our environments and our bodies.

The levels we are exposed to clearly depend on many lifestyle factors. The life-stage we are at can be crucial to our health and that of our children, particularly unborn babies in utero and new born babies given bisphenol A feeding bottles.

Bisphenol A Facts

- BPA exposure is bad for snails, causing them to produce so many eggs that they burst

- BPA is in seawater and has been found in many marine species that are eaten by humans

- BPA is in the epoxy resin coating used in some tin cans so that the food inside can be heated to temperatures high enough to kill any bacteria without the metal of the can contaminating the content. Consequently, many canned foods are now contaminated with bisphenol A instead

- The vast majority of babies feeding bottles are made of BPA

- Women tend to have higher concentrations of bisphenol A than men; this may be due to differences in exposure or metabolism between the sexes

- Although not without controversy, various strands of research have implicated BPA in breast cancer, male reproductive system defects, miscarriage, immune system defects, polycystic ovarian disease and recent research has revealed a possible link to diabetes, insulin resistance and obesity (6 - see ref. on page 126)

- Put more simply, bisphenol-A seems to have a complex and potentially insidious effect on the human endocrine system, with a possible knock on effect on the immune system. There are also indications that very low concentrations can produce negative health effects – especially when it comes to foetal sensitivity (exposure of the foetus in the womb through the placenta)

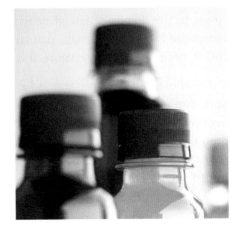

- As with phthalates, pregnant women are especially advised to minimise their exposure and, post-natally, to ensure that baby feeding bottles are either not polycarbonate or if they are that they are discarded every three months or as soon as any scratches or other signs of wear and tear occurs.

What products contain it and how does it get into me?

- Bisphenol A is used to make plastic food containers including the ones used in microwaves, water bottles, the coating of the insides of cans and other food containers, in DVDs, mobile phones, electrical appliances, baby feeding bottles, sports equipment, spectacle lenses, some car parts, medical equipment, refrigerator shelves, eating utensils, dental sealants, flooring, paints and adhesives. It's also present in certain pesticides and flame retardants, and is used as a stabiliser in rubber chemical and PVC

- Ingestion is a major exposure route both because bisphenol A is often in contact with food and drinks, particularly water and babies' milk formula and is known to leach from products that contain it – and because polycarbonate plastics degrade over time

- Inhalation from house dust

- From mother to child through the placenta and breast milk.

Alternatives

- Minimise in-take of canned foodstuffs, especially those with a high fat content

- Use glass bottles instead of polycarbonate, especially for repeated use

- Don't have white fillings at the dentist, better still pursue good dental hygiene so as to avoid fillings in the first place

- Use glass instead of bisphenol A baby bottles

- Do not microwave in plastic

- For picnics and food on the move try to use metal and glassware and paper cups and plates rather than plastic.

48

5. FORMALDEHYDE

What is it and what threat does it pose?

For many people formaldehyde conjures up memories of sitting at big wooden school benches looking at a splayed out rat on the biology teacher's dissection board, trying not to breathe in the horrible smell. So, it will come as a surprise to find out that the same pungent chemical can be found extensively in home environments, in carpet backing, curtaining, flooring, domestic cabinets, as well as in a range of products that have an even more intimate relation to our bodies such as lipstick, toothpaste and soft drinks. It is most commonly found in many brands of 'diet' soda where it is a breakdown product of artificial sweetener (see below). Formaldehyde is a very volatile organic chemical. Even quite low-level exposure can affect the mucous membranes of the eyes, nose and throat causing burning and watering of the eyes, burning of the nose and throat, coughing and difficulty in breathing. Higher and prolonged exposure can result in skin and lung allergies and it has been strongly linked to asthma and various cancers.

Formaldehyde is produced worldwide on a large scale – in its form as urea formaldehyde resin it is extensively present in particle-board, plywood and other pressed wood products. MDF, or medium density fibreboard – that stalwart of the DIY-er – contains the highest concentration and emits the most formaldehyde into the air. Formaldehyde is strongly associated with so-called 'sick building syndrome' because of its extensive use in various building products and the tendency it has to 'off-gas' – which means it significantly releases as a gas, especially when a product containing it is new and in conditions of warm temperatures and high humidity. These releases can continue for as long as a year after installation and vary in concentration according to heat and humidity.

Embalmers use formaldehyde to preserve dead bodies and, strangely enough, this 'preservative' function is also employed by the cosmetics industry in many shampoos, hand-washes, bubble baths and other personal grooming products of an aqueous nature. Exposure to formaldehyde in the general environment also comes from vehicle exhausts, smoke (tobacco, coal and wood), dust and vapours off-gassing from construction, insulation and interior decorating materials.

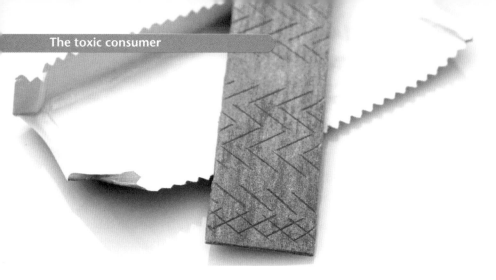

Formaldehyde Facts:

- Aspartame (found in many table-top artificial sweeteners, diet drinks, diet food, chewing gum etc) breaks down into wood alcohol (methanol) which further breaks down into formaldehyde in the body which, if regularly present, can cause gradual, and eventually, severe damage to the neurological and immune systems

- Formaldehyde used to be used as an insulating foam but was banned in the early eighties because of its toxicity to human health

- It mixes easily with water, but not with oil or grease, and is often used as a cheap preservative for aqueous personal grooming products like shampoos, hand-washes and even baby bubble bath

- Levels of formaldehyde in outdoor air are generally low, but higher levels can be found in the indoor air of homes

- Contributes to 'sick building syndrome'.

What products is it in and how does it get into me?

- Common sources of exposure include particle board, MDF and similar building materials, carpets, paints and varnishes, foods and cooking, tobacco smoke, and the use of formaldehyde as a disinfectant

- Ingestion and inhalation are the most common exposure routes.

Alternatives

- Try to install hardwood or other natural flooring instead of carpets or PVC

- Choose toothpaste and other personal grooming products that do not contain formaldehyde as a preservative

- Ideally choose alternatives to MDF or particle board for kitchen cabinets etc, but if you do use them then don't cut them at home without a mask and good ventilation. Seal them with a low VOC sealant as soon as possible (see Chapter four on Indoor Pollution)

- Don't allow smoking in the home or the car since cigarette smoke contains significant amounts of formaldehyde (along with many other chemicals)

- Use low VOC paints, varnishes and other wall and floor substances

- Drink water and fresh juices rather than 'diet' drinks with aspartame.

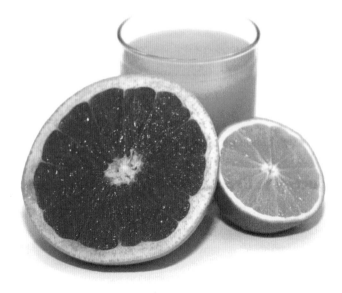

6. SYNTHETIC MUSKS

What are they and how do they get into me?

The human body apparently smells a little musky, especially when aroused, which is why the small but potent gland of an otherwise innocuous miniature deer that lives high in the Himalayas became so plundered by mankind in our efforts to smell even 'muskier' and be more attractive to other humans. The story goes that Henry VI was so addicted to the smell of natural musk that he died through over-indulgence of his habit of sniffing it.

International protection efforts and modern chemistry came to the rescue of the musk deer when it became a protected species and chemists managed to isolate its primary odorous element, muscone, in 1926. Synthetic musk was born. Real musk is still produced, but only about 700 pounds of it per annum and it costs roughly three times its weight in gold. In dramatic contrast, around 800 metric tonnes of synthetic musk are produced annually, and for a bewildering range of uses. It's generally used in a 'fixative' as opposed to an aromatic role to make things like air fresheners, fabric conditioners and body lotions as well as actual perfumes, smell 'better' for longer. The high molecular weight of synthetic musks combined with their ability to blend easily with other aromatic ingredients, make the olfactory potency of those ingredients more penetrating, more enduring and deeper. So something doesn't have to smell 'musky' if it has synthetic musk in it – the musk element is more likely to be there to amplify another smell, like violet, rose or lavender. Except in certain, single note perfumes where the bald intention is to try to create a sexy musky scent. Strangely enough it is usually perfumes aimed at women that try to mimic the smell that derives from a sac that nestles next to the male musk deer's prostate gland.

On a molecular level, smell actually does touch your nerves and it is quite common for synthetically scented products to have acute adverse effects, triggering headaches, migraines, asthma, allergies and causing irritation to the eyes, nose and throat. Strong scents are often described to be 'choking' and 'eye-watering' and some people are clearly far more sensitive than others to these negative effects. Others can stand in a perfume hall all day squirting passers-by

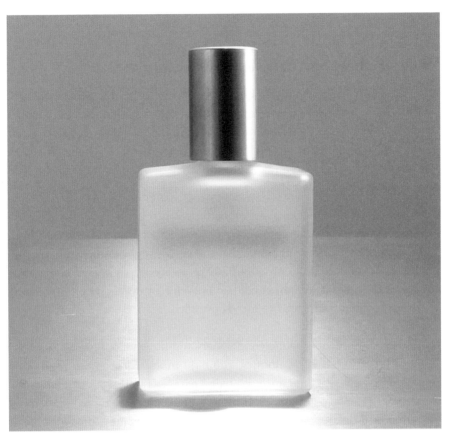

while suffering no apparent ill effects. However, synthetic musks are both bioaccumulative and persistent in the environment and some are known to be toxic, like Musk Ambretta and Musk Xylene for example, which have already been discontinued. Others previously considered only mildly toxic are being re-evaluated in the light of some fascinating, if worrying, new research. There is a possibility that polycyclic musks, the most common by far, may act as 'toxic enhancers' by debilitating the cells' natural ability to defend against other toxic substances. If this is the case, considering that the plethora of products that contain synthetic musks also often contain other hazardous chemicals like parabens, phthalates and bisphenol A, then their toxic consequence could prove to be far more enduring and widespread than the smells they are there to prolong and intensify.

Musk facts

- There are three main groups of synthetic musks: nitro musks, polycyclic musks and macrocyclic musks. Musk xylene (a nitro musk) poses a particular problem, as it is a widespread contaminant of the environment. The polycyclic musks are thought to be less environmentally-damaging than nitro musks, but they are also persistent, bioaccumulative and toxic to reproduction. Both have been highlighted as possible carcinogens. Macrocyclic musks are currently being investigated as possible substitutes for the other two musk groups

- Levels of polycyclic musks have been seen to be increasing in concentration in some human breast milk samples

- Recent research shows that both nitric and polycyclic musks may compromise the body's xenobiotic defence system: the basic defence mechanism that allows the body to pump toxic substances out at a cellular level

- A number of nitro-musks, a family of inexpensive synthetics used widely for decades, have actually been taken off the market in recent years because of their "photo-toxicity" – they become poisonous when exposed to the sun

- The almost magical property of synthetic musks to enhance and prolong the smell of whatever it is added to explains its success across the spectrum of fragrance chemistry, musk is to fragrance what MSG (Mono sodium glutamate) is to Chinese food

- A lot of people are allergic to perfumes, this can manifest in various ways, as skin reactions, headaches and migraines, general nausea and irritation of the mucous membranes

- AHTN& HHCB are the most common polycyclic musks – 95% of the EU market.

What are they in and how do they get into me?

- Synthetic musks are almost as ubiquitous as phthalates and parabens and are often found in the same products, especially those we use for personal grooming and skin care. Wherever there is 'parfum' there is usually synthetic musk, and as well as the obvious, perfume, cosmetics, hair shampoos, conditioners and styling treatments, body washes, shaving foams etc, they are also found in detergents, clothes conditioners, air fresheners, bin bags, children's toys, scented candles, toothpaste, sweets and almost every imaginable consumer product that manufacturers think can be made more appealing by adding fragrance, including chewing gum and ice cream

- Our exposure is typically through the skin and via inhalation of 'fragranced air', although a certain amount will be through ingestion of fragranced foodstuffs, toothpaste and cosmetics such as lipstick, lip balms and other products applied around the mouth area.

Alternatives

- Either don't use perfume or use less, it will more than likely repel as many people as it attracts and understand that in the vast majority of cases it's utterly synthetic and laden with chemicals

- Avoid gimmicks like 'fragranced bin liners' (just empty the bins regularly)

- Be aware of the heavy fragrance added to hundreds of everyday consumer products while shopping and always opt for non-fragranced or fragrance-free versions

- Use small quantities of essential oils if you need to add some smell to your products. Places like Neal's Yard sell them and can advise on appropriate quantities and combinations

- Ventilate the home rather than use so-called 'air fresheners'. In the loo, strike a match to disperse bad smells and install an extractor fan

- Avoid perfumed children's toys.

7. PARABENS – ARE YOU BEING WELL PRESERVED?

What are they and what threat do they pose?

Parabens have been used as preservatives since the 1920s, to prevent the growth of bacteria in a wide range of consumer products including a variety of foods and pharmaceutical drugs. Their most prevalent use, however, has been as a preservative in facial and body cosmetics, skincare products, shampoos and conditioners, sunscreens, underarm products (antiperspirants and deodorants), colognes and perfumes, and soaps. They are cheap to produce and hard to 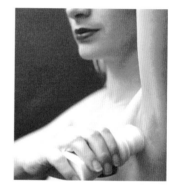 avoid: the most widely used preservatives worldwide. Their rapid excretion from the body (in both human and animal testing) has led to a general assumption that their toxicity is of no real concern. However, more recent research has raised concerns that further assessment of parabens is required. This is based on over a dozen scientific studies indicating that several types of parabens can bind to the oestrogen receptor and cause oestrogen-like responses. Other research showing that endocrine-disrupting chemicals can cause side effects at extremely low doses calls into question the safety of parabens, given their common presence in so many products that we use everyday and often several times a day. The recent discovery of parabens in breast tumours has led to speculation that they may be implicated in breast cancer (particularly since their action as an oestrogen mimicker has been shown in research). The fact that most breast tumours occur in the part of the breast nearest to the armpit has led to further theories that parabens in underarm deodorants may be a culprit. This hypothesis has drawn currency from the fact that breast cancer is more common in the left breast, the idea being that because most people are right-handed they apply more paraben-containing product to the left armpit. Although an interesting theory, it is entirely unsubstantiated and much more research needs to be done. As a precautionary measure, it is probably worth avoiding paraben-containing deodorants and to avoid application of under arm products or other skin products immediately after shaving.

Paraben Facts

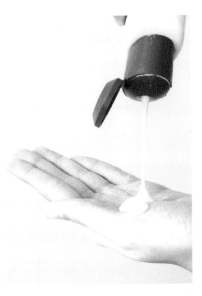

- The four parabens in common use are: methyl-, ethyl-, propyl-and butyl-parabens and most products will contain 2 or more of these chemicals as part of their preservative system

- Paraben Allergic Hypersensitivity is a form of allergic contact dermatitis and affects a minority of individuals. It seems to result from repeated applications of relatively low concentrations of parabens in products ranging from cosmetics, personal grooming products, foodstuffs and even children's gel-like play products like 'slime'. Some cases have even been recorded of severe genital eczema occurring in men after they have used condoms impregnated (sic) with benzocaine and parabens!

Where are they and how do they get into me?

- Cosmetics, shampoos, body creams, shaving creams, some deodorants, pies, some children's gel-like play stuffs, condoms, pharmaceutical products, nail products, baby lotions, shampoos and bath products

- Exposure through the skin is of much more concern than ingestion since the body's digestive system easily breaks parabens down

- Parabens have been found in breast milk, in the blood and other body tissues and they can cross the placenta and enter the foetus in utero

- Although they are metabolised relatively quickly, like phthalates, our almost constant exposure to them means that they are generally in the body

- Some Japanese research on methyl-paraben found that it did not metabolize in the strateum corneum, the outermost layer of the epidermis, and suggested that its presence accelerated skin aging.

Alternatives

- Paraben-free options do exist and are generally found in health stores or in 'green' ranges available in selected supermarkets. Always check the label first. Generally speaking the four main parabens are listed in the list of contents

- Simple emollients such as aqueous cream tend to work just as well as complex, highly fragranced, additive laden 'premium beauty' products and it's worth remembering that good diet, lots of water and exercise will do more for your skin than any amount of face cream

- A number of manufacturers are responding to consumer concerns over parabens and are developing preservatives made entirely from naturally occurring ingredients – for example, a Canadian product called Naturbak. However, given the shelf life requirements of many consumer products, it is difficult to find all-natural alternatives that will preserve things for the durations generally required. One solution is to have products with a shorter shelf life, but this tends to diminish profitability so is unattractive to most companies

- Choose ranges such as Jo Wood Organics or Ren since these go out of their way to avoid synthetic chemical ingredients and still manage to produce a high end, effective range of products with good distribution

- Generally streamline your personal care approach, use fewer products and choose those with more natural ingredients.

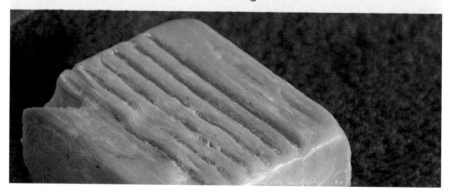

58

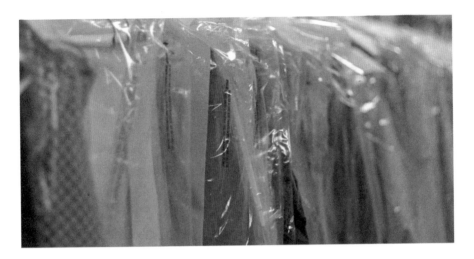

8. PERCHLOROETHYLENE or 'PERC'

What is it and what threat does it pose?

The phrase 'being taken to the cleaners' refers to the bad business practices of the original 'dry' cleaners who would return garments smelling of petrol and expect their customers to accept them. When you get your dry-cleaning back from today's chemical processes you might be forgiven for thinking that nothing much has changed. Frankly, most dry-cleaning smells pretty bad, and comes back swathed and enclosed in a layer of flimsy plastic that serves to preserve that acrid, unpleasant smell in your clothes, in your closet and ultimately, in you too. Ironically it is usually our most delicate, natural-fibre clothing that tends to get the chemical clean – silk blouses, wool suits and coats and so on. 'PERC' or perchloroethylene is a chlorinated solvent and the most common dry-cleaning solvent in use. Originally developed as an industrial de-greaser, it's been the staple of the dry-cleaning business since the thirties. But, in the light of recent evidence as to the toxicity of 'PERC', the dry-cleaning industry is increasingly having to seek greener, cleaner alternatives. PERC is a very volatile organic compound, a hazardous air pollutant and groundwater contaminant and causes effects in humans ranging from dizziness and nausea to liver and kidney problems – it is neurotoxic if inhaled in large quantities and is listed as a probable carcinogen.

'PERC' facts

- Occupational exposure to PERC has been implicated in higher incidences of cancer of the oesophagus in several US studies

- The majority of the dry-cleaning industry is keen to hang on to PERC – it is the solvent of choice because of the cost implications of changing and because it is such an effective product. But at what cost to health and the environment?

- In 2003, Southern Californian 'air quality' officials voted to impose America's first ban on PERC, the vote requires the phasing out of all PERC dry-cleaning in Los Angeles by 2020

- PERC is used by approximately 80% of European dry-cleaners

- PERC has been used as a general anaesthetic agent because at high concentrations it produces loss of consciousness.

Where is it and how does it get into me?

- The greatest exposure of PERC to consumers occurs when people live in buildings with dry-cleaning facilities, wear recently dry-cleaned clothes or store such chemically laden garments in their wardrobes and drawers

- PERC is also found in some spot or stain removers, specialised aerosol cleaners, some water repellents, suede protectors and wood cleaners. Check the contents label

- The primary exposure route is via inhalation of fumes, but because of its persistence as an environmental pollutant it is in the water we drink and the food we eat too

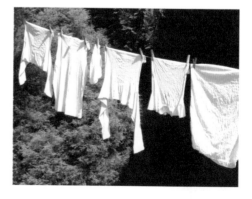

- PERC can also enter the body through skin contact, although this is less common.

Alternatives

- Don't buy 'dry-clean only' clothing in the first place

- Seek out less toxic cleaning methods. In the UK, the Johnson Group (who own Sketchleys and 'Jeeves of Belgravia') is switching to the GreenEarth cleaning system which uses silicone-based Siloxane D5. However, it is far from proven to be environmentally sound since it is manufactured using chlorine and may be responsible for dioxin emissions. Research is currently being done on its potential toxic fallout

- Use the new computerised 'wet' cleaning machines which are able to control agitation and humidity levels to reduce the chance of shrinkage

- Liquid Carbon Dioxide is being adopted by some drycleaners as an alternative to PERC

- If your clothes have been cleaned using a PERC process then remove the plastic and air thoroughly before bringing them into the home or putting them away in your wardrobe.

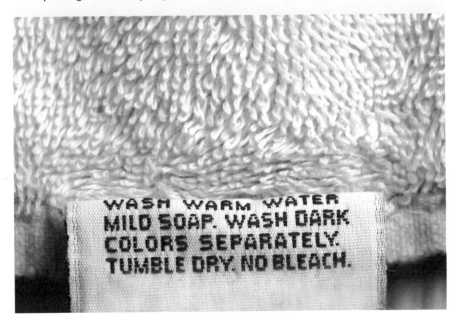

9. ORGANOTINS

What are they and what threat do they pose?

Organotins are chemical compounds based on tin with hydrocarbon substituents. They are used as stabilisers or catalysts in PVC, silicones, polyesters and polyurethane, as well as in glues and wood preservers. One compound, tributyltin

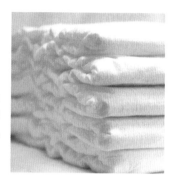

(TBT), was widely used as an anti-fouling paint on boat hulls, to stop barnacles and other foulants attaching themselves to the metal hull, until it became clear that it was having a devastating effect on the marine life left in its trail. It was shown to have serious endocrine-disrupting effects on a variety of marine life. Perhaps most dramatically evidenced in the poor female dog whelk, whose exposure to TBT resulted in them developing penises and in some case actually exploding because the eggs they were producing had nowhere to go. It may therefore come as something of a surprise to learn that the same chemical has been found in a curious range of consumer products that includes baking paper (now withdrawn), plastic toys, paddling pools as well as in things which came into rather more intimate contact with the body such as insoles, socks, nappies and the crotch padding of cycling shorts. There are some concerns that the chemicals, which are persistent and bioaccumulative, can enter the body and attack the white blood cells on which the human immune system depends. Other concerns include the fact that tributyltin (TBT), a chemical compound that is known to disrupt sex hormones, has been found in disposable nappies on sale in the UK. If a baby wears an average of five nappies a day, he or she could be in contact with up to 3.6 times the World Health Organisation's estimated tolerable daily intake. Although its transdermal uptake has not been established it is known that the chemical can be absorbed through the skin. The fear is that the chemical may be absorbed into the body and disrupt the child's sex balance since very small levels have been shown to be disruptive to endocrine function. Although many manufacturers claim to have removed TBT from their nappies, it is worth checking because it is can be there almost accidentally as a by-product of plastic polymerisation during the manufacturing of the polyurethane membrane on some nappies.

ORGANOTIN facts

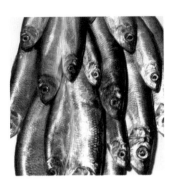

- TBT is a classic gender bending chemical in nature, causing snails and female dog whelks to change sex

- TBT is found in fish all over the world and in marine mammals including seals, dolphins and whales which are unable to expel it from their bodies.

Where are they and how do they get into me?

- As well as in nappies, organotins are found in various sanitary protections since they are made in a similar way, in inflatable beach toys like water wings and beach balls, in PVC flooring, in the 'plastic' heat-transfer printing on football shirts and other clothing, in sports shoes, household paints. They are also commonly used as fungicides in children's socks

- Organotins are found extensively in house dust and exposure can be through inhalation or transdermally

- Another major exposure route is through ingestion of contaminated seafood

- Because organotins exhibit PBT characteristics, they are also widespread environmental contaminants and are in our food and water.

Alternatives

- Use washable nappies – they are better all round
- If you use disposables select eco-friendly, biodegradable options
- If you do choose the bleached, additive-enhanced, mass-market options then try to select brands that actually state that they do NOT have TBT in (Some carry the tag 'certified TBT free)
- Reduce PVC products and don't buy children's beach toys made with TBT
- Don't buy clothing that promises 'added fungicide' or similar labelling.

10. TRICLOSAN

What is it and what threat does it pose?

A product of modern day hygiene obsession, triclosan is the chemical made by man to make as many things as possible anti-bacterial and anti-microbial. It gets added to handwashes, toothpastes, deodorants and impregnates plastic chopping boards, bin bags, plastic kitchenware and cleaning cloths. It's also a close relation of dioxin which happens to be one of the most potent synthetic animal carcinogens ever tested. Dioxin causes damage to development, reproduction, and the immune and endocrine systems at infinitesimally low doses (in the low parts per trillion). Toxicological studies have not been able to establish a "threshold" dose below which dioxin does not cause biological impacts. But that's dioxin. Triclosan manufacturers state that their product is safe, that it biodegrades and is not bioaccumulative. These claims are doubtful given that it has been detected in freshwater streams, in sewage effluent and in fish from lakes affected by domestic sewage input. It's also been found in human breast milk and breaks down in sewage treatment works to 'methyl' triclosan which is even more bioaccumulative and if you add sunlight to triclosan in sewage it can convert to dioxin itself. Another bad characteristic of triclosan is that when combined, from a soap or detergent that it's been added to, with chlorinated tap water it produces chloroform. On top of all that, in its original bug-killing function it is probably contributing to the increased antibiotic resistance of bacteria in the environment which has health implications for us all. Its scatter

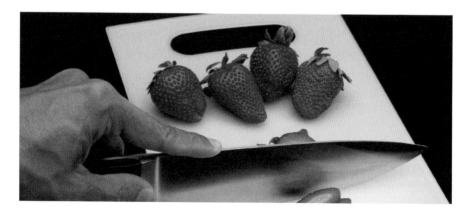

gun, undiscriminating and take-no-prisoners action on bacteria means that it also kills the 'friendly' bacteria that occur naturally in our bodies and environment and which aid our digestion, metabolism and general eco-systemic balance. Insufficient testing has been performed on the wider potential consequences of triclosan, but the singular facts of it's chemical 'lineage', its presence in breast milk combined with the relative superfluity of its function means that it is best avoided wherever possible.

Triclosan Facts

- It has been estimated that triclosan's bioaccumulation factor is high enough to classify the chemical as "very bioaccumulative" according to the UK Government's Chemicals Stakeholder Forum's criteria for chemicals of concern

- The United States Environmental Protection Agency (EPA) has registered it as a pesticide and gives it high scores both as a human health risk and as an environmental risk

- Anti-microbial formulas and disinfectants can also cause genetic mutations resulting in drug-resistant bacterial and mutant viruses, producing new strains of harmful microbes for which the human immune system has no defence

- One of triclosan's manufacturers proudly lauds it as the 'aspirin' of anti-bacterial agents and boasts that it stays on the skin for hours after washing as a 'secret protection'!

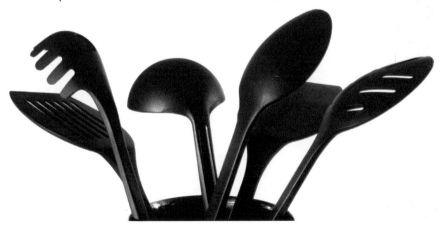

65

What is it in and how does it get into me?

- Soaps, deodorants, toothpastes, mouthwash, anti-acne and foot-care products, plastic cutting boards, plastic kitchen utensils, children's toys, socks, underwear, school uniforms and bedclothes

- Ingestion from mouth-washes and tooth-pastes as well as contaminated food-stuffs

- Absorption through the skin from soaps and skincare products where it is used as a preservative, often alongside parabens.

Alternatives

- Several retailers are already phasing out triclosan

- Sweden no longer sells products that unnecessarily use triclosan and Norway is considering a complete ban

- Be wary of clothing or bedding advertised as anti-bacterial, they probably are impregnated with it

- There is really no reason to use products that contain triclosan in domestic environments, just adopt a good and regular cleaning routine.

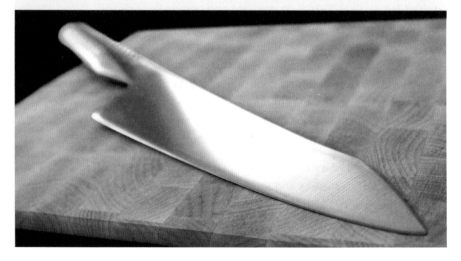

PLUS! The best of the rest...

Clearly, there are many more than ten chemicals, out of the thousands that are in common consumer goods, that potentially pose a risk to human health. Most everyday cosmetics and personal grooming products contain a potent cocktail of parabens, phthalates, toluene (see below), formaldehyde plus a whole host of other chemicals, but its difficult, and highly litigious, to start extrapolating without adequate research data. However, detailed below are some other common toxic chemicals that are commonly used despite big questions being raised as to their safety with regard to human health, wildlife and the environment.

Alkylphenols, especially nonylphenol – high production volume chemicals used for over forty years as detergents, emulsifiers, wetting and dispersing agents. Although they were phased out as domestic detergents in the UK in 1976, they are still extensively used in consumer products, in shampoos, cosmetics and spermicidal lubricants. They are not readily biodegradable and are known aquatic pollutants. The European Parliament wants to restrict nonlyphenol as a 'priority hazardous substance' on account of its persistence, bioaccumulation, aquatic toxicity and endocrine-disrupting potential.

Sodium lauryl sulphate (SLS) – a very common chemical found in shampoos, hair conditioners, toothpaste, body washes and bubble baths. SLS started out as an industrial de-greasant and garage floor cleaner. When applied to human skin, it has the effect of stripping off the oil layer and then irritating and eroding the skin, leaving it rough and pitted. It can have terrible effects on the eyes, causing cataracts in adults and is capable of inhibiting proper eye development in children. And it can cause mouth ulcers. But it makes products foam up better so they seem super soapy, and that's why SLS is added to common consumables. Best to check the label and select SLS-free products. If in doubt, keep well away from the eyes and mouth.

Toluene has a variety of uses. In consumer products, it's often added as a solvent in paint, adhesives and some detergents and is regularly added to hairsprays, shoe polish, nail polish, perfumes and cosmetics. When used by solvent abusers (glue sniffers), it can cause irreversible hearing loss, central nervous system and brain damage from excessive exposure. In terms of day-to-day exposure, it is most likely to be absorbed transdermally by using personal care products that contain it or through inhalation of indoor air that is contaminated with it from nearby solvents. Chronic low-level exposure to toluene can cause irritation of the upper respiratory tract and eyes, sore throat, dizziness, and headache. Reproductive effects, including an association between exposure to toluene and an increased incidence of miscarriages have also been noted however these studies are not yet conclusive due to many other variables.

Methylisothiazolinone (MIT) and methylchloroisothiazolinone – regularly used as an antimicrobial agent or biocide in personal care products such as shampoos and hand lotions. MIT and related compounds kill harmful bacteria that like to grow near moisture or water and are also often found in water-cooling systems. Recent laboratory-based research has revealed that even a 10-minute exposure at a high concentration proved lethal to the nerve cells. This chemical is being used more and more extensively, yet there have been no neuro-toxicity studies in humans to indicate what kind of effect it may have despite clear indications that it could have neuro-developmental consequences.

Mineral Oil – like 'baby oil' is a petroleum by-product that coats the skin like plastic, clogging the pores. It can interfere with the skin's ability to eliminate

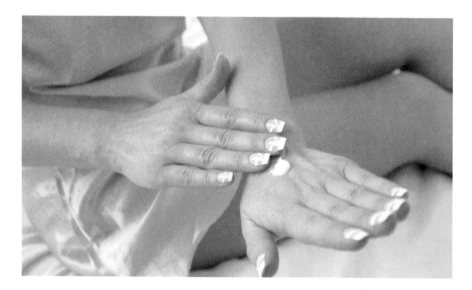

toxins, thereby promoting acne and other disorders and slowing down skin function and cell development which results in premature aging. Any mineral oil derivative can be contaminated with cancer causing PAHs (polycyclic aromatic hydrocarbons- see below)

Polycyclic aromatic hydrocarbons – PAHs

Where there's smoke, there's usually some polycyclic aromatic hydrocarbons in the air.

PAHs are ubiquitous environmental contaminants formed during the burning of organic substances such as wood, coal, oil, gas, rubbish and tobacco. Initial concerns about PAHs focussed on their carcinogenic properties but more recent research has implicated them in endocrine disruption, toxicity to reproduction and their ability to suppress immune function. There is also evidence that their effects increase synergistically when combined with other pollutants. In terms of consumer products, they are found in processed food and produced by tobacco smoke, fireplaces, woodstoves, home barbecuing and the charring and burning of food in conventional ovens. But even if you don't smoke, barbecue, burn the dinner or have an open fire, PAHs will be present in your home as a result of prolonged industrial activities.

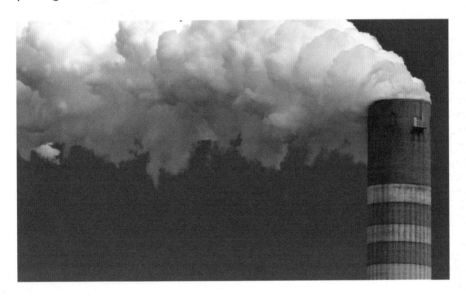

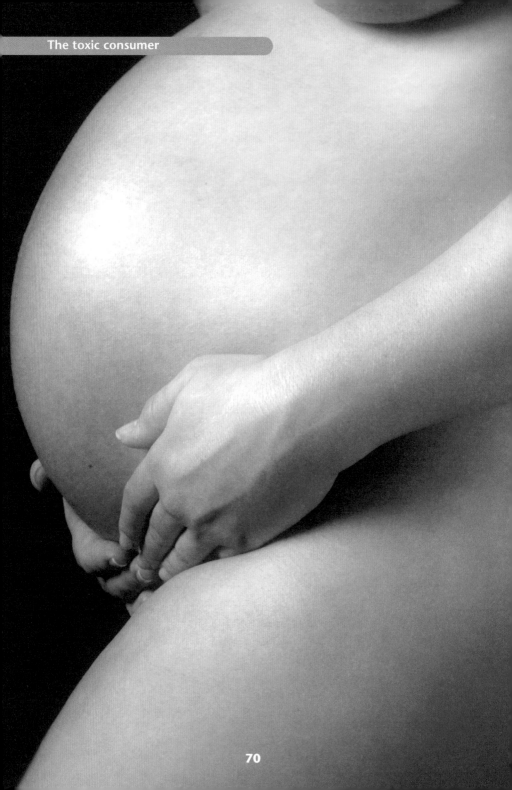

3

Sensitive subjects

There are many variables with respect to the effects toxic chemicals have on human health and well-being. A major factor is that we are all more sensitive to certain substances at particular stages of life than at others. For example a baby developing in utero is the most sensitive, most vulnerable and the least able to protect itself from harmful chemicals. Endocrine-disrupting chemicals (EDCs), commonly termed hormone disruptors, are particularly worrying here. Put very simply, much of the assessment of 'safe' levels of exposure relates to averages based on the effects of toxic chemicals on the healthy, fully grown adult male which are then scaled down to account for effects on children, women and babies. A lot of these assessments are made with regard to workplace and occupational exposure as well and do not really address personal or family exposure via the domestic environment. The inadequacy of this approach is the subject of much current research: especially with regard to chemicals known to have an effect on hormones, because hormones have an indefinable number of roles according to the metabolic process involved, the sex and life stage of the subject.

Another important variable in considering the relative safety of substances is that some individuals are far more sensitive than others to the effects of certain toxic chemicals. One person may develop an allergic reaction or a migraine after exposure to a particular product, such as a perfume, while another may experience no symptoms at all. In extreme cases a small minority of people develop a condition known as 'multiple chemical sensitivity (MCS)' where a range of allergies and intolerances seem to occur with low-level chemical exposure. This condition can be extremely debilitating because it is nigh on impossible to avoid MCS-causing chemicals and still live a 'normal' life.

This chapter covers first, the crucial issue of foetal sensitivity and the special vulnerabilities of the child and secondly, the issue of why some people are more sensitive than others. It underlines, once more, why a precautionary approach and minimising exposure to toxic chemicals is the only sensible option.

A question of dose

Back in the 16th century, a controversial Swiss physician, Paracelsus, coined the phrase 'the dose makes the poison'. The idea being that the higher the dose of any particular chemical, the greater its toxic effect will be on living organisms. His ancient words still inform much contemporary toxicological assessments of substances. However recent research into endocrine-disrupting chemicals has shown that this is not always the case. A far more accurate assessment of the situation is to say it is the dose **plus** the timing of the exposure to it that makes the poison. Furthermore, scientists have discovered that in some instances extremely low doses of certain compounds can induce stronger negative or toxic responses and be more dangerous than higher doses: even when the test organ-

isms are at the same life stage. In some cases, there are no effects at higher doses because after a certain level of exposure there may be negative feedback – essentially cutting off any response. This is known as the 'Low Dose phenomenon' (ie. low doses are more dangerous than higher ones), or the upside down 'U', where the reaction increases with dose up to a point and then falls off – hence the shape of this on a graph with dose measured along the bottom and response up the side (see page 74). This fundamental paradigm shift in knowledge of the action of toxic

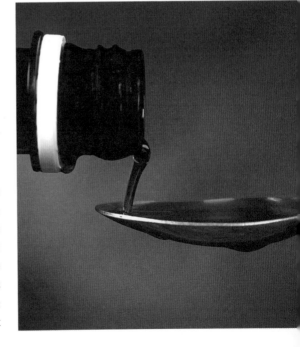

73

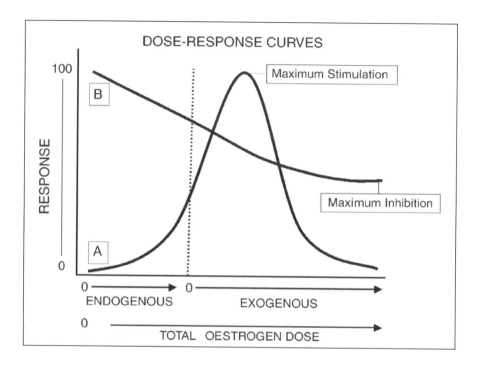

chemicals is especially the case with those that affect the hormone system and throws into doubt much conventional wisdom about 'safe' levels of known endocrine disruptors in particular. This is especially so during most vulnerable periods of development, eg. the foetus in utero.

A question of balance

As touched on in Chapter One, the endocrine system is one of the three major systems of the body and operates in intimate relation to the immune and nervous systems. The three must work in perfect harmony in order for us to be well and to feel well. The hormones produced by the endocrine glands are powerful biological messengers responsible for orchestrating development and behaviour from the earliest time of differentiation in utero through to old age. Their action is mostly taken for granted and goes unnoticed but the hormonal ravages of puberty, experienced to a greater or lesser extent by us all, are a clear testament to the power of our hormones. Another occasion when hormone effects are apparent is when the endocrine system is undermined by an external factor, such as chemicals which have the ability to mimic or disrupt naturally occurring hormones.

The endocrine system is a complex, finely-tuned, subtle and highly-evolved messaging system on a molecular level and its disruption can have far reaching consequences on both physical and mental health. A number of synthetic chemicals are known to have the capacity to interfere with the normal function of the natural chemicals of the body – the hormones – either by blocking, imitating or having an opposing effect. Some of the most studied endocrine-disrupting chemicals (EDCs) to date have been high production, high volume man-made chemicals such as bisphenol A and phthalates. In some cases these have been shown to have a feminising effect either by mimicking the female hormone (oestrogenic effect) or stopping the action of the male hormones (anti-androgenic effect) and are implicated in a range of conditions from arrested sexual development in the male to accelerated sexual development in the female. Research indicates that effects include lowering of sperm counts and rising rates of hormone-related diseases such as breast and testicular cancer. Other synthetic chemicals that are beginning to receive more attention are those suspected to disrupt thyroid and pancreatic function, such as BFRs and perfluorinates. EDCs are being linked to rising rates of diabetes and other metabolically linked disorders.

Generally, incidences of non-infectious diseases in children in the developed world are rising: conditions such as asthma, allergies, diabetes and various auto-immune disorders. In some populations, there are also rising incidences of reproductive system defects and other anomalies such as a general lowering of sperm counts and earlier onset of puberty. Since immune response and primary sexual development is determined during antenatal and early postnatal development, much research has been focussed on this sensitive stage. Endocrine-disrupting chemicals and the 'low dose' phenomenon has special ramifications for the foetus, babies and young children, as it does for chemical legislation which has a responsibility to protect our young from toxic chemical interference right from the moment of their conception.

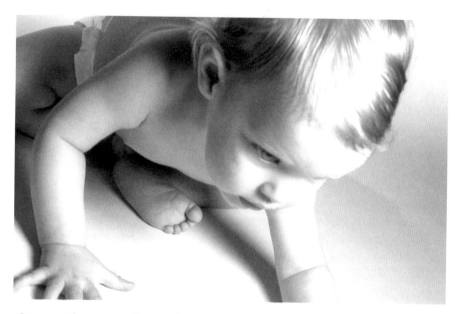

Questions of scale and timing

In assessing the toxic effects of chemicals, children and babies cannot be regarded simply as scaled down versions of adults. Physiologically they are very different and they live very differently too

- They eat more food per pound of body weight, hence can take on a greater volume of toxic chemicals pound for pound

- Food stays in the baby's/child's digestive tract for longer meaning longer potential absorption times to take up toxic chemicals ingested in food. For example, a young child will absorb 50% of ingested lead compared to 10% for adults

- A high percentage of the diet of babies and young children is cow or breast milk which makes for a higher relative fat intake and higher proportions of lipid-soluble chemicals such as PBTs as detailed in Chapter Two

- The blood-brain barrier, which limits the ability of the majority of chemicals to pass into the lipid content of the brain, is in gradual development during early childhood so throughout this time, there is higher potential risk of exposure from neuro-toxic chemicals

- Babies and children breathe more rapidly, so are proportionally exposed to more air pollutants

- They have significantly different ratios of body fat and water content to adults and a higher skin surface to body weight ratio. Also their skin is more permeable so they are prone to higher dermal absorption

- Because of higher dermal absorption, it is worth considering time spent in the bath since water does contain a variety of contaminants, in addition to whatever bathroom products are added to the water

- They live differently, spending most of their time closer to or on the ground so that their exposure to the various chemicals found in house dust, in carpets and on flooring is greater

- They constantly put things in their mouths

- They generally absorb chemicals more easily, process them more slowly and eliminate them less efficiently

- A lot of children's clothes, including school uniforms and pyjamas, are treated with perfluorinates (to make them crease resistant and/or water and stain resistant), brominated flame retardants (to protect them from fire risk), phthalates (often in those shiny plastic cartoon transfers on t-shirts/pyjamas etc.) and organotins (such as TBT, often impregnated into kids' socks as a fungicide.) These chemicals are rarely flagged up on any labelling attached to the clothes. Taken all together, they represent quite a chemical cocktail for the child

- Protective mechanisms available to the adult such as DNA repair or the blood-brain barrier are not fully functional in the newborn or young child, and yet, they are exposed to the same or sometimes higher levels of toxic chemicals

- For older children approaching puberty, a time of raging hormones, mood swings, confusing feelings, spots, sometimes acne and fundamental physical and mental change, the last thing they need is any more chaos. However there is an increasing amount of research which shows that adolescence is often coming preternaturally early, kicking off auto-immune disorders, diabetes, exacerbating allergies and other problems.

EXQUISITE FOETAL SENSITIVITY

The reason that the timing of exposure to endocrine-disrupting chemicals is so crucial for the foetus and young children is that the body's systems are most sensitive when they are under construction. During the early stages of development important events are occurring all the time, providing many small pockets of opportunity when the developing organism can be extremely sensitive to hormone-disrupting chemicals, such as during the formation of the testes. This is known as 'exquisite sensitivity' because of the almost unimaginably small amount of hormone that a foetus can be sensitive to. It has been shown to be as tiny as one part per trillion (a million times lower than one part per million). Any toxic chemicals that can mimic hormones need to be considered in the same light, ie. potentially toxic in infinitesimally small quantities.

A cautionary example of the power of some EDCs is shown by Diethylstilbestrol (DES), a synthetic oestrogen prescribed to pregnant women in America between the late 1940s and the early 1970s. It led to many reproductive abnormalities in both male and female offspring, many of which did not become apparent until the offspring themselves reached puberty and beyond. Subsequent experiments on rats demonstrated how DES exposure at particular stages of foetal development led to reproductive system damage similar to that exhibited by the human victims. DES was a pharmaceutical product that superseded bisphenol A as the synthetic oestrogen of choice until its devastating consequences became apparent many years later.

Meanwhile bisphenol A, as detailed in Chapter 2, has found its way into common use in a whole range of everyday consumer products. Since the effects of many of these chemicals may be additive, exposure to a range of endocrine-disrupting chemicals at low levels may have a similar effect to a higher level of exposure to one chemical. It's a distressing fact of contemporary life that regardless of lifestyle or location, the expectant mother will inevitably pass on a significant part of her toxic body burden to her offspring, both via the placenta and through breast milk. The placenta, essentially a barrier designed to protect the foetus, is robbed of this function when it comes to toxic chemicals of a low molecular weight that dissolve readily in fat. And while breast is still considered best, it's sadly not as good as it used to be because of the accumulation of chemicals in breast milk.

- Very low levels of chemical interference can be catastrophic at very sensitive developmental stages

- Once across the placenta the hazardous chemicals can mix into the amniotic fluid which is constantly sipped and swallowed by the foetus. Then it can be absorbed by the digestive tract or skin, thereby leaving the maternal circulation and entering the foetal circulation

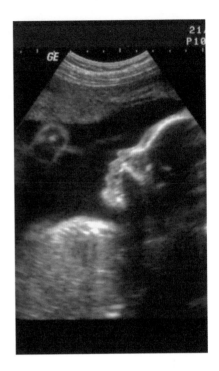

- The developing foetus lacks subcutaneous fat reserves which can act as a buffer to lipid-soluble chemicals in older children and adults. Fat-soluble chemicals are more likely to end up being stored in foetal tissues that have high fat content such as the brain

- The cells that produce sperm and eggs (germ cells) start to develop in the foetus and, in the case of males, mature during puberty. Chemicals can damage the germ cells which may result in the adult's fertility being harmed and congenital defects in them or their offspring. More and more research is indicating that the male system is particularly vulnerable to chemical interference in utero

- The embryonic period, weeks 3-7 following conception, is a period of rapid development: early formation of organs and major systems and exquisite sensitivity

- Premature infants are particularly at risk of increased early exposure to phthalates because of the PVC tubing and other medical devices that they get hooked up to in intensive care

- Sudden post-natal loss of weight is not recommended since this will mobilise the mother's fat reserves and release toxicants into her blood and into breast milk. Slow, gradual weight loss is recommended.

Testicular dysgenesis syndrome (TDS) hypothesis

The TDS hypothesis is used to describe disorders that affect many males and are either apparent at birth or show up in adulthood. They are thought to be linked to abnormal events occurring in utero. The disorders evident at birth include failure of testicular descent into the scrotum (cryptorchidism) and incidences where the urethral opening is wrongly located on the penis (hypospadia). In many cases both of these disorders require surgical correction. In adulthood, incidences of low sperm counts/infertility and testicular germ cell cancer are becoming increasingly common in young men. These disorders are considered to be interconnected. It is generally thought that abnormal testicular cell development plus interference with sex steroid hormone action (ie. androgens and oestrogens) are probably involved and that genetic, lifestyle or environmental factors may induce the syndrome. It's a hypothesis that is the cause of much concern and has been written up extensively in many respected medical journals, including The British Medical Journal and The Lancet.

The development of the testes occurs almost entirely during early development in utero where cells called the 'Sertoli' cells, responsible for producing sperm in later life, begin to differentiate. Exposure to oestrogen concentrations at this time has been shown to reduce the number of Sertoli cells that are produced and this could be one explanation for lowering sperm counts. There is also evidence to suggest that abnormal germ cells, formed in early development, are responsible for most testicular cancers in later life.

- Several studies have documented that men with undescended testis and/or hypospadias are significantly over-represented among patients with testicular cancer

- There is evidence that men who later develop testicular cancer have a lower proportion of male children (offspring sex ratio) than other men

- Although the endocrine-disrupter hypothesis is considered both relevant and plausible at the time of writing relatively few chemicals have been closely examined for their potential effects on hormone activity

- The seriousness of the problem is highlighted by recent health statistics from Denmark where trends in reproductive diseases, including testicular cancer, are showing a worrying increase. Almost 1% of (mostly young) men are treated for testicular cancer, an amazing 5.6% of schoolboys have undescended testes and almost 1% have penile abnormalities when they are born. Furthermore over 40% of young adult men have subnormal sperm counts (Skakkebaek and Sharpe).

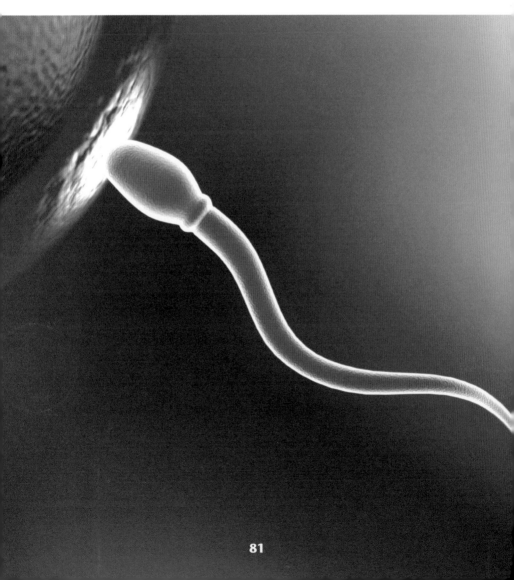

Multiple chemical sensitivity (MCS) – over-sensitive or hyper-sensitive?

A sensitive subject in itself – and more so in the US than the UK – a lot of people dismiss MCS as a catch-all excuse and stigmatise people who claim to suffer from it as time wasters, hypochondriacs and so on. There is a general reluctance on the part of the medical profession to 'legitimise' it as an illness because there are so may other factors that could contribute to the symptoms associated with it, which are various and include the following:

- burning, stinging eyes
- sore throat, cough
- wheezing, breathlessness
- extreme fatigue/lethargy
- headache/migraine
- poor memory & concentration
- light & noise sensitivity
- digestive problems

- runny nose (rhinitis)
- sinus problems
- nausea
- muscle & joint pain
- vertigo/dizziness
- skin rashes and/or itching skin
- sleep disturbance

What is certainly true is that some people do have much more extreme reactions to toxic chemicals in consumer goods than others, in rare cases to such an extent that they may not even be able to walk down the detergent aisle in a supermarket without their eyes streaming and skin starting to itch. Why this is the case is difficult to pin down although there are plenty of theories. The standard industry canard that all these conditions are psychogenic or psychosomatic is increasingly being queried by researchers in the field. It is worth noting that, until relatively recently, antibody-mediated conditions such as various allergies and asthma were considered to be psychosomatic until the real cause was identified. Along the same lines, there is research that shows that some of the reactions grouped under the umbrella term MCS may find a medical explanation in the form of certain enzyme deficiencies. This would explain why a chemical

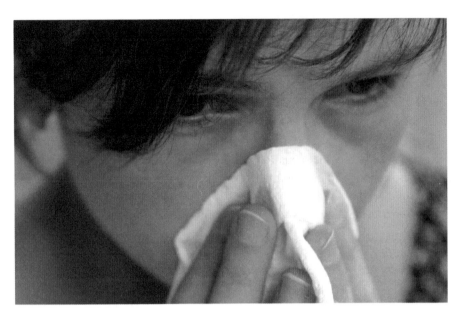

trigger can cause debilitating symptoms in one person whereas another will experience no discernible effects. It is clearly important to recognise biochemical individuality/variability of tolerance and genetic difference affecting our ability to detoxify certain chemicals from the body. Something like lactose intolerance is often confused with an allergy to milk products, whereas actually it is a deficiency of an enzyme which breaks down lactose in the body. So if it is the case that a certain percentage of the population lack the enzyme to break down organophosphates for example, as is hypothesised by several researchers into Gulf War Syndrome, then this has ramifications for the producers of such chemicals.

Another factor to consider with respect to individual chemical sensitivity is the process of sensitisation, the process by which the body becomes highly reactive to a particular substance after repeated exposure to that substance. An initial exposure can cause the body to mount an exaggerated immune response and since the immune system has its own form of memory, after sensitisation has occurred it will overreact every time the allergen or antigen is present in the body thereafter. This can happen to allergens in nature such as pollen or particular foodstuffs (peanuts and strawberries are common examples). It can also

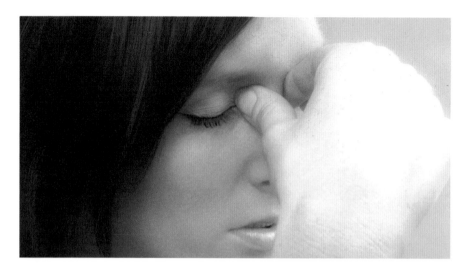

happen from exposure to toxic chemicals. Occupational sensitivities are quite common where chemical agents are part and parcel of daily use, for example vehicle spray painters have very high rates of occupational asthma (90 times the national average). Hairdresser, barbers and beauticians have high rates of contact dermatitis (up to 16 times the average) and painters and decorators often have respiratory and skin conditions from prolonged exposure to the volatile organic compounds and solvents they use (government occupational health statistics 2004/2005).

Not necessarily as debilitating, but far more common, are adverse reactions to synthetic fragrance, with even the briefest exposures capable of bringing on headaches and other unpleasant symptoms such as fatigue or difficulty in concentrating. The adage 'one man's meat is another's poison' seems to be particularly relevant when it comes to perfume – one person will splash it on all over and love it whereas it'll leave the next person gagging and running for the door for some fresh(er) air. In all of these cases, avoidance is the best policy. Unfortunately, this is increasingly difficult when so many common products contain such a wide range of chemicals. The task of identifying exactly which of these triggers the reaction is made even harder by a paucity of labelling. Again, self-education and awareness of which products cause adverse reactions are important to help minimise exposure to those chemicals that simply don't agree with you.

4

Indoor pollution and how to reduce it

Pollution is a word we tend to associate with grimy city roads, exhaust fumes, industrial plants billowing noxious smoke and catastrophic events such as oil spills. We do not generally associate it with the cosy indoor environment we lock ourselves up in every night. Yet pollution levels inside the home can be as high, often much higher, than levels outside even for inner city dwellers. Furthermore, the type of pollutants found in the home can be very different to those we are exposed to outdoors but they still pose a significant health concern. Since we spend a lot of our time inside, at home, in the car or workplace it is important to know both the sources of, and how to reduce, indoor pollution levels in your indoor environments.

The modern love affair with wall-to-wall fitted carpets, double-glazing, central heating and heavy domestic insulation all contribute to keeping the indoor air inside. Good for keeping out the cold but not so appealing when you consider that there may be a heady cocktail of volatile organic compounds and other chemicals off-gassing from paints, other floor and wall coatings, particle board (chip board, MDF etc), carpeting, various plastics, the flame retardants in soft furnishings, electronic products and gizmos, phthalates in PVC flooring and so on. Plus there will be sporadic surges after cooking with non-stick cookware, a mad half hour with super strength cleaners, or spraying air fresheners or stain repellents. Even the effects of a steaming hot day can make toxic chemicals more volatile than usual. And then there are all the 'on-body' pollutants to take into account too – all those personal grooming products with their various blends of chemicals given direct access to your skin. While there are clear energy saving benefits to double glazing and home insulation it is absolutely essential to have outdoor air flowing and circulating in the home so the concentration of any contaminants in the indoor air can be reduced. Having a house full of chemically laden fixtures, furnishings and products in a near-airtight environment makes for a very unhealthy living situation.

A quick and easy way to reduce indoor pollution then, in the short-term, is to open a few windows and ensure that your home gets plenty of ventilation and

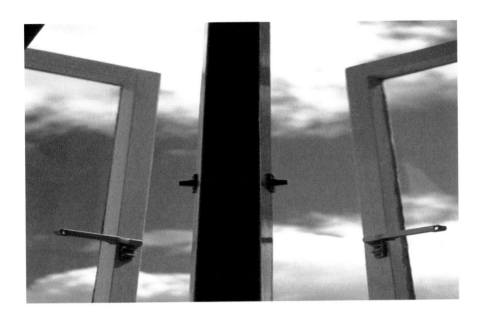

thorough air circulation. However even this simple solution can be compromised if you shut everything up overnight for fear of intruders, to keep energy costs down or because you are going away on holiday. Window locks can be fitted to allow a small amount of air in, or bars can be installed that pull back in the daytime. Clearly there are exceptions to wanting the outside air inside: if you live next to a waste incinerator, or a huge industrial plant or in a basement flat next to a busy road for example. In these situations you probably do want to keep the outdoors outside and have to make your indoor environment as fresh and hazardous-chemical free as possible. Whatever your situation, generally it's worth making a step-by-step assessment of the toxic potential of your indoor environments. Then draw up a short-term strategy for products you can either do without or can find less toxic alternatives for; a medium-term strategy for reducing your exposure to the more volatile organic compounds and other toxic chemicals in your home and a long-term strategy for when you can make bigger changes such as replacing flooring or furniture, or even moving home.

If you've read this book up to this point, you'll have a pretty good idea of which chemicals are found where in consumer products and in the domestic environment. This chapter is a guide to the most common sources of indoor pollution and offers suggestions for alternative products.

Everyone's home environment is different and it's a good idea to make an educated assessment of the health of yourself and others that live with you. If there's a high incidence of headaches, dizziness and general inexplicable fatigue, or if people simply report feeling better when they leave the home, indoor pollution may be a problem and steps should be taken to reduce it. Also, some individuals may feel worse after using certain cleaning products or spraying air freshener or perfumes. Often we put these adverse reaction down to other lifestyle factors, 'some virus or other', working too hard or too many late nights, when it may well be pollution at home. Symptoms such as headaches or eye, nose and throat irritation, allergies and asthma are acute symptoms and are more or less immediate reactions to contaminants. There are many other more chronic effects that can result from long-term, consistent exposure. These may lead to respiratory disease, heart disease, immune disorders, reproductive defects and cancer. People will react in a number of ways to different toxic chemicals; babies and children being especially vulnerable.

House dust

The presence of most of the toxic chemicals mentioned in this book in house dust is a good indicator of the indoor levels of contaminants. It also puts paid to various manufacturers' claims that dangerous chemicals are bound into products and therefore do not present an exposure threat. In a major analysis of house dust performed by Greenpeace in 2003, it was found that all dust samples (from 100 homes in ten different regions across the UK) contained brominated flame retardants, phthalates and organotins in addition to a whole range of VOCs and other solvent and plastic additives. Exposure to dust in the home represents a significant direct exposure route for humans and is of particular concern with respect to children. The received wisdom that house dust is just an accumulation of dead skin cells and random dirt particles is no longer accurate and, given its toxic content, care should be taken when disposing of it from dustpans or vacuum cleaners. As an indicator of the scale of contamination of our homes, dust is a lowly but important signifier and while we may be motivated to vacuum and dust more often in the light of these findings, in the long-term we need to insist that manufacturers use less leaky and less toxic chemicals in products destined for our home environments.

Toxic shag

Fitted carpets have become by far and away the most popular floor covering in the UK and much of America. While they have considerable thermal and acoustic advantages as well as the all important comfort and convenience factors, there are a number of reasons to consider other flooring options. Although they have been embraced as an easy, hassle-free flooring solution, apart from harbouring dust and its concomitant mites, carpeting is often heavily treated with brominated flame retardants, stain resistors (perfluorinated chemicals), anti-microbial treatments (organotins), formaldehyde (usually in the glue backing) and various pesticides – all of which may off-gas or leach into the domestic air. Furthermore the shag-pile tends to attract and harbour airborne particles including pollutants from VOCs, synthetic fragrances, paints, cleaning products plus all the pollutants brought in from outside on the feet. Aside from the common toxic chemicals detailed in this book, old carpets have also been found to contain high concentrations of heavy metals such as lead, cadmium and mercury, polyaromatic hydrocarbons and PCBs. Researchers at the Manchester Asthma and Allergy Study Group reported in The Lancet that "environmental manipulation", including removing carpets from infants' bedrooms, reduced symptoms of asthma and allergies in high-risk babies. Carpets also collect pet allergens, heavily implicated in childhood allergies and asthma, which are then spread from place to place on pet-owners' clothes.

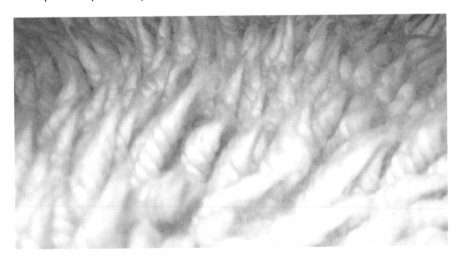

If you do have fitted carpets throughout the home it is important to keep your home well-ventilated and the carpet well-vacuumed (making sure not to over-fill the bag if it's that type of vacuum cleaner!) It's important to make sure that your vacuum cleaner is up to the job. If it's not a well-sealed unit then it's liable just to kick up and redistribute the dust back around the room and into the air at the same time. Carpet can hold up to 8 times its own weight in dirt, so clearly the deeper the shag – the more toxic it can be. Some newspapers have even dubbed carpets 'the toxic sponge'. If you are thinking of fitting carpets, or even having rugs, try to have them aired before being installed and avoid gluing them down. Stapling is a better option. Choose a naturally flame retardant product like tightly woven wool with a natural backing such as jute or a hemp and cotton mix, containing natural stain inhibitors such as lanolin from fleece. In the bigger environmental picture, carpets and rugs such as these are also biodegradable at the end of their domestic service.

PVC flooring

If you have wall-to-wall carpets and PVC flooring everywhere else you really do have one of the most toxic combinations underfoot. It is especially important to review these floorings if you have young children because of their susceptibility to asthma and allergies and their closeness to ground level. PVC flooring contains phthalates, chlorinated paraffins and possibly lead or tin compounds as

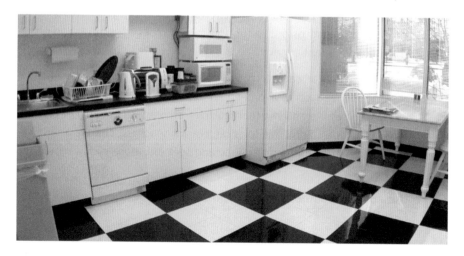

stabilisers. The phthalates leach into house dust, into the air and transfer to the water used to clean them. PVC is associated with increased risk of asthma since a Nordic survey linked exposure to chemicals used to soften PVC to inflammation of the airways. Many countries are already restricting PVC in public buildings because of health and environmental risks, yet there is a trend in the UK for schools to install both carpets and PVC flooring because of cost and durability. Sweden does not allow fitted carpets in schools, public buildings or offices. Linoleum, wood, rubber, and other alternatives are just as hard-wearing and as easy to maintain as carpet and PVC but much less likely to accumulate allergens. Furthermore, dioxin may be created in the manufacture of PVC, and may be created again if it's destroyed by incineration.

Healthier flooring options

- Wood, from sustainable forests, if you select wood laminates insist on low or zero emitting boards

- Natural linoleum – naturally anti-bacterial, antistatic and resistant to fats and oils, long lasting, low maintenance and made from renewable materials

- Try Bamboo – it's a very renewable resource, but check on preservatives and look out for the boric acid content

- Natural rubber – another good renewable resource, good durability and sound absorption, although avoid rubber flooring with chlorinated content

- If you like rugs or carpet try to select those with vegetable fibre content as they won't have been sprayed to protect against animal-borne diseases like anthrax (particularly from eastern nations) or with other pesticides. Look out for sisal, coir or seagrass, choose a tight weave for natural flame retardance and seek out those with a natural backing

- Use a doormat at the front door and try not to wear shoes around the home.

Toxic slouch and slumber

The simple enjoyment of snuggling up in bed, or on the sofa of an evening may be compromised if you realised just how much toxic chemical content can be nestling there in the fibres just inches from your nose. Bedding, soft furnishings, mattresses, cushions, pillows can be heavily treated with a range of chemicals, from the ubiquitous flame retardants through stain guards, organotins and even synthetic musks. Wrinkle-free bedding may contain formaldehyde, the 'ticking' of your mattress may contain PVC, and the whole surface might contain perfluorinates for water and stain resistance (especially children's mattresses). Labelling of 'contents' is often wholly inadequate and the only way to ensure a chemical-free or reduced product is to buy from a source advertising its status as such. Since we spend such a long time in bed and often in intimate skin contact with bedding materials, it is worth investing in combinations of natural products, organic cottons, latex and natural wool. Natural fibres are more tightly woven, more naturally flame retardant and give off far less mattress emissions than those made with polyurethane foams and vinyl coverings. Polyester sheets and night wear, apart from the alarming habit they have of sparking up as you clamber into them, are also not very healthy sleeping partners.

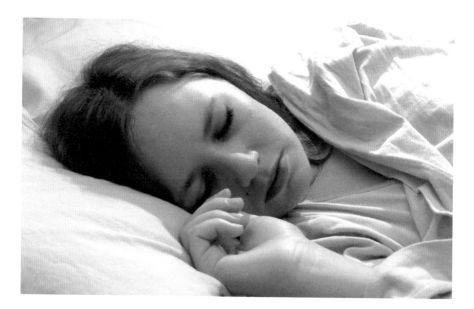

Safe sleep tips

- Choose organic cotton mattresses and bedding that allows you and your skin to breathe easily wherever possible

- Buy from manufacturers that have found alternatives to brominated flame retardants, such as IKEA

- Avoid gimmicks such as 'fragranced' pillows or other bedding

- Don't have bedding dry-cleaned, but if you absolutely have to and can't find a PERC-free service then be sure to air it well before using it

- Keep your bedroom well-aired and as free of consumer products such as computers, televisions, fragranced candles, carpeting and perfumed products as possible

- Be especially vigilant about the content of your baby's cot and mattress. This is the last place to compromise since the baby's airways are smaller and more vulnerable to allergens and toxic chemicals

- If you are unsure as to the content of new mattresses, let them 'off-gas' in a well-ventilated room before sleeping on them.

HI –tech & toxic

Modern technology has delivered us a whole range of electronic ways to be entertained and to communicate while at home. TVs, DVD players, VCRs, PDSs, MP3s, games consoles, stereo systems, plasma screens, laptop and desk top computers, home movie projectors, mobile phones and wireless phones are all commonplace domestic gadgets, often regardless of socio-economic background. They are a mass of plastic casings, semi-conductors, super-fast processors and liberal quantities of chemicals including the ubiquitous phthalates, formaldehyde and brominated flame retardants. These chemicals off-gas into the indoor air the longer they are turned on and the hotter they get, especially if the products are new. They also leach out of the products into house dust that settles on objects and on flooring and inevitably circulates in the air as we move about disturbing the dust. In the broader environmental context, the disposal of defunct or simply unwanted 'e-waste' is a huge problem. Much of the content cannot be disposed of safely or recycled. Pressure needs to be put on the manufacturers of these products to develop safer, more sustainable and less toxic alternatives, but meanwhile:

- Try to purchase from manufacturers that are committed to researching and using greener, cleaner chemicals in their products like Ericsson, Dell and Philips (do your research since this list will be expanding all the time)

- Choose metal or wood casings over plastic wherever possible

- Turn electrical goods off when not in use

- Don't let them over-heat

- While electrical goods are still new make sure to keep the rooms you are using them in well-ventilated

- Keep these products to a minimum. Resist the temptation to upgrade your phone/MP3 player/PDA every few months – newer products 'off-gas' more than older ones and its environmentally irresponsible to frequently discard so many items.

Dirty but clean

Cleaning products can be pretty dirty. Take the black scum that collects in your washing machine powder and conditioner receptacles for example. There are multiple chemicals that go into the various high power de-greasers, drain de-cloggers, oven cleaners, floor cleaners and conditioning fluids, and often there is strong synthetic fragrance to cover up the horrible chemical smell that would otherwise prevail. Countless individuals are sensitive to cleaning products, coming out in lumps and bumps or experiencing irritated mucous membranes, headaches and nausea. The simple answer is to completely refine the products you use to clean and freshen your home. Try to use less products, select 'green' brands, use more of your own muscle and appreciate that the more combinations of products you regularly use the more complex the toxic chemical cocktail

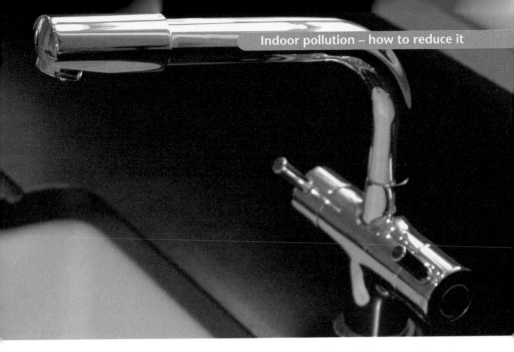

you are going to be exposing yourself and those that live with you to. Cleaning agents emit volatile organic compounds (VOCs), including formaldehyde. They also regularly contain phthalates, synthetic musks and triclosan – chemicals that can pose a wide range of hazards to human health.

What might be lurking in the products under your sink?

- **Oven cleaners** contain powerful alkaline corrosive agents such as sodium hydroxide or potassium hydroxide. A single exposure can severely burn the skin and damage the eyes. Aerosols are worse since a mist of the caustic chemicals can drift on to skin, eyes and sensitive lung surfaces. Most oven cleaners do warn that they can burn skin and eyes and that fumes and vapours should be avoided. So if you can't avoid using them do take their warnings seriously. Ensure proper ventilation and wear a mask and rubber gloves

- **Washing powders** (especially the 'biological' kind) are often based on a corrosive alkaline chemical called sodium carbonate, also found in dishwasher powders. This can cause adverse effects in people with sensitive skin. Even wearing the washed clothes can trigger an effect, which can be followed by an immune reaction producing an itchy rash that can spread across the body and last for several months to a year. Some sufferers claim that simply walking down a supermarket aisle stacked with boxes of biological washing powders can make them feel itchy

- **Shoe polish** may contain a solvent called nitrobenzene. As well as providing that distinctive smell, it's also a suspected human carcinogen that affects the central nervous system producing fatigue, headache, vertigo, general weakness and, in some cases, severe depression. It reacts with alcohol so best not to polish your shoes while having a beer! Shoe polish can also contain methylene chloride – a known animal and suspected human carcinogen

- **Drain clearer** often contains the same caustic chemicals as oven cleaner – (sodium hydroxide and potassium hydroxide) or sulphuric acid. All very toxic and if you can't avoid using them, then follow the safety instructions religiously

- **Bleach** contains sodium hypochlorite, which irritates and corrodes mucous membranes, causing pain and vomiting if swallowed. Breathing in fumes causes coughing and choking and may cause severe respiratory tract irritation. Go easy with the spring-cleaning and perhaps wear a shower cap while you're at it – exposing the scalp to vapours containing sodium hypochlorite has been known to cause acute, toxic alopecia, as the vapour can alter the hair structure

- **All-purpose cleaners** typically contain a scary combination of detergents, grease-cutting agents and possibly solvents and disinfectants, plus one or more of the following – ammonia, ethylene glycol, monobutyl acetate, sodium hypochlorite and trisodium phosphate. They can cause anything from mild to extreme irritation to the skin, eyes, nose and throat. Chronic irritation can occur after repeated use

- **Metal polish** – buffing up the family silver can provoke headaches, nausea, dizziness, hallucinations and, at extreme levels, coma. A typical solvent in metal polish is toluene which has been linked in human studies to reproductive and developmental disorders. High and repeated exposure during pregnancy has been associated with nervous system defects, urinary tract and gastrointestinal problems, and raised miscarriage rates. So snap on the gloves, open the windows, and don't do it very often

- **Air freshener** – a misnomer with bells on! Some of these products mask unwanted smells with synthetic fragrance, others work by deadening our own sense of smell so although the original bad smell is still there, we just can't smell it any more. Lots of the aerosol varieties contain isobutane, butane and propane which may produce simple asphyxia, with symptoms such as dizziness, disorientation, headache, excitation and central nervous system depression, and anaesthesia. Try opening some windows and sprinkling some essential oils around instead

- **Washing-up liquid**, like all detergents, contains chemicals called surfactants that lower the surface tension of water, making it runnier and more able to 'be wet' and so better able to clean. They also encourage water loss from the skin, leaving it dry and irritated. Healthier vegetable-derived surfactants are easily available but the petrochemical versions prevail because they are cheaper. Wear rubber gloves, if you have a dishwasher don't touch the powder and better still use an eco-friendly range.

- **Don't** mix different household cleaners or solvents together. This can turn your kitchen into a dangerous chemical experiment

- **If you want to avoid chemical cleaners** try using the following basic, natural cleaning agents: **white vinegar** (it doesn't smell and mixed with water it cleans windows, glass, tiles and surfaces), **baking soda** (mixed with water it becomes an all purpose cleaner for sinks and baths and can be sprinkled over carpets as a deodoriser), salt (for scouring pots and pans), **lemon juice** (as a bleach in laundry, mixed with vinegar to de-clog sinks), and **olive oil** (mix with vinegar to polish furniture). Check out 'Clean and Green – The Complete Guide to Non-Toxic and Environmentally Safe Housekeeping by Annie Berthold Bond (Ceres Press, 1994)

- **Choose 'green' cleaning ranges** wherever possible.

Kitchen checklist

- If you use non-stick cookware then keep temperatures low and ventilation high. Throw the pans away if there are any signs of surface degradation

- Use glass and ceramic food containers rather than plastics – especially avoid soft plastics and food being in contact with one another

- Keep cleaning products well away from foodstuffs

- Don't use triclosan impregnated cutting boards or other kitchen products.

- Avoid having MDF or chip-board units in the kitchen if possible – especially newly installed. If you do then give them a good chance to air properly before putting food back into your kitchen

- Use extractor fans to take away smoke and cooking smells – don't use kitchen air fresheners

- Don't microwave in plastic.

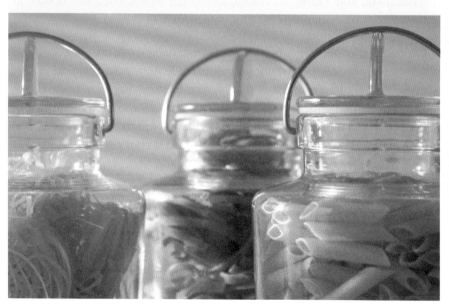

Do-it-yourself home improvements

Whether you are donning overalls and breaking out the workbench yourself or employing the professionals, home decorating can cause a sharp spike in levels of indoor pollution, both at the time and for a good while afterwards depending on the products used. There are a lot of reasons to be precautionary when engaged in these kinds of activities and it is best if you can seal off the areas being renovated, or temporarily move out altogether if it's an option.

- Up to 90% of the internal surface area of a building could have a synthetic petro-chemical covering. These coverings will commonly contain numerous defoamers, stabilisers and sundry other chemicals whose effect on health is largely unknown

- Try to avoid using jigsaws or other cutting gear on particle-board or MDF at home without excellent ventilation and some form of breathing protection. Better by far is to measure it all up and get it cut accurately to your own spec at the timber-yard. If you do cut it at home, it's best if people aren't living there at the time and that you seal it as quickly as possible to stop it off-gassing into your home. Untreated, freshly cut MDF is not a safe option, in the author's opinion, unless it's a formaldehyde-free version

- Paint and other decorative finishes made from natural raw materials are a real substitute for today's conventional paints made from petrochemical derivatives. They are simple to use and apply and because they do not use petrochemical ingredients, they bring a number of environmental and health benefits. Natural paints also offer high standards of protection, longevity and ease of use. They are also more 'breathable' and do not attract as much dust

- Conversely, as well as many synthetic solvents being classified as carcinogenic, the volume of them in the air during application can exceed recommended levels by up to seven times. As a result, professional painters are prone to suffer from dermatitis, bronchitis, asthma and nervous system disorders. Petrochemical paint manufacturers promote their water-based paints as a less toxic alternative to their oil-based ranges but check them out thoroughly first. They may actually contain more chemicals than the oil-based type they are intended to replace. Vinyl resins, such as those found in conventional emulsion wall paints, can damage lungs, liver and blood, are skin irritants and possible carcinogens

- Seal off-gassing sources (such as particle board and MDF) with impermeable barriers like a low VOC varnish or latex paint

- Allow gases from new furnishings and building materials to be given off in storage for a few weeks or even months before you bring them into your home. If this is not possible, try to increase the ventilation in the affected area(s) by opening windows and doors for as long as possible

- Buy paints, cleaners and solvents in small quantities – just enough for what you need. Recycle old or no longer wanted tins and bottles and, if you can, store leftover products in a separate building like a garage

- Keep lids on tight.

On-body pollutants

These are the creams, lotions and other potions that we smooth over our skins, massage into our hair, pat around our eyes, brush on our lashes and rub on our lips, that we roll or spray under our arms, bathe in and that some people occasionally even douche with. The average lady at her 'toilette' can use twenty products or more in one sitting and re-applications of some of them may happen several times a day. And men are catching up fast, and some really do splash it on all over – often with quite overwhelming results going out with hair like meringue peaks and leaving a potent blend of synthetic-macho fragrance in their wake. Most generally available personal care products contain a lot of chemicals. Even ones that carry words like 'organics', 'fruits of the forest' or some other natural-seeming name are more likely to be fruits of the laboratory and organic as in organic chemistry. These chemicals get inside us and we do not know the extent of their individual, let alone combined, action.

- Common chemicals in everyday personal care products: **phthalates** * **parabens * triclosan** * mineral oils * FD & C colours * diazolidinyl urea * propylene glycol * polyethylene glycol * diethanolamine * lanolin *

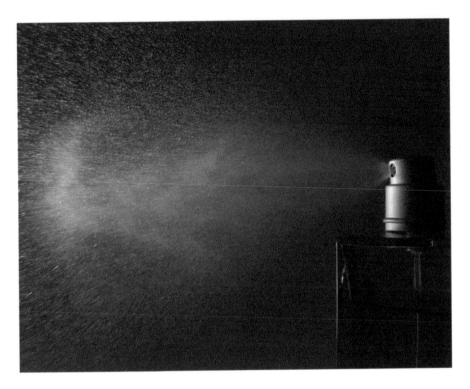

triethanolamine * tetrasodium EDTA * polysorbate * imidazolidinyl urea * dimethicone * phenoxyethanol * cetearyl alcohol * cetyl alcohol * cocamide DEA * cocamidopropyl betaine * glyceryl stearate * emulsifying wax * capric/caprylic triglycerides * olefin sulfonate * myristamine oxide * octyl methoxycinnamate * stearalkonium chloride * petrolatum * monoethanolamine * **synthetic fragrances (musks)** * **sodium lauryl sulphate**

- Choose petrochemical-free ranges such as Ren and Dr Hauschka

- Streamline your personal care routine to use fewer products and start to work on your beauty regime from the inside out too. Drink lots of water and get plenty of fresh air and exercise!

- Try to cut down on cosmetic use. In many cases it's tantamount to covering your skin in a very thin layer of plastic

101

- Avoid products that contain synthetic fragrances or 'parfum'

- The cosmetics and personal grooming industry is not regulated like the food industry yet a lot of the content can be absorbed transdermally. So as you scan a content list like the one above perhaps ask yourself the question: Would I eat this? And if you wouldn't, then perhaps think twice about putting it on your skin – it's the largest organ of the body and a lot of absorption occurs through it

- Screening the sunscreens – a lot of new sunscreens and some new cosmetics contain a chemical (titanium dioxide) as a nanoparticle and there are concerns about its ability to pass through the skin or be inhaled. Studies have shown that inhaled nanoparticles can be much more toxic to health than micro particles of the same chemical (see Chapter 6).

In-car pollution

In many ways the car is a microcosm of the home with its leather or fabric uphol-stery, various kinds of electrical gadgetry, lighting, carpets, phones, in-car entertainment systems and lots and lots of plastic. Almost everything you get exposed to in the home will also be in the car: flame retardants in abundance, perfluorinates to resist staining, formaldehyde in the carpets, phthalates and bisphenol A in the plastics. So what exactly is that new car smell? The answer is a complex mixture of volatile organic compounds (VOCs), primarily alkanes and substituted benzenes along with a few aldehydes and ketones. Nearly every solid surface inside a vehicle is a fabric or plastic that is held together in part by various adhesives and sealers. Off-gassing of the residual solvents and other chemicals from these materials leads to a dilute mist of VOCs floating about in the passenger compartment. So when you push the internal air circulator button to keep out all that nasty outdoor pollution, have a thought for what's in the air inside the car already. A Japanese study revealed that the 'new car smell' could contain up to 35 times the healthy limit set for volatile organic chemicals in Japanese cars in their domestic market, making it an experience akin to glue-sniffing. The chemicals found included ethyl benzene, xylene, formaldehyde and toluene used in paints and adhesives. The study reported that it took three years for the level in cars to fall below the limit set for vehicles by the Japanese health

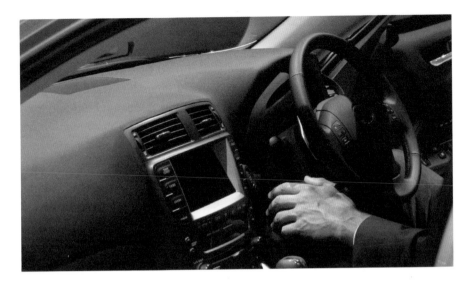

ministry: a limit set in response to an increase in the number of car owners suffering from sick building syndrome. Official figures are not yet available in the UK but suffice to say ventilation is once again key, and sucking air through the chemically-infused plastic vents is probably not as effective as just having the windows open a little.

- Clearly, that new car smell isn't good for you and many people experience an otherwise inexplicable nausea when inside a very new car, so it's important to air it as much as possible. It can take about six months for a 'new car' smell to fade and the related higher health risks to subside. Even if a car has 'off-gassed' substantially a steaming hot day can revitalise all those VOCs, so try not to leave the car in direct sunlight. If you do then it's good to air it well with all the windows and doors open before you get in and drive off

- A far more cost-effective and healthier option is to buy a second hand fuel-efficient car rather than a new one, since the chemicals will have had a chance to off-gas and the indoor pollution levels will be much lower than with a machine straight off the production line

- Keep abreast of new products on the market since car manufacturers are slowly getting more tuned into making greener, cleaner machines and some brands will have lower chemical content than others

- There are no government restrictions on in-car pollution levels and for a lot of manufacturers their main aim is to keep the VOCs low enough to prevent fogging of the windows with no real thought as to the hazards of such high chemical content in an enclosed space

- Some car dealers even sell 'new car smell' fragrance sticks, to keep that fresh-from-the-showroom aroma going on indefinitely!

- Pregnant women and young children should avoid spending extended time in brand new cars

- If you feel dizzy or slightly 'high' while driving, pull over, get out of the car and get some fresh air before proceeding.

Understanding that your indoor environment may be significantly polluted, and how, is the first step to improving your domestic situation. The benefits will be apparent in the short, medium and long term and while not many of us can afford to change all our flooring and furniture and so on in one go, we can all improve our indoor air quality significantly just by introducing better ventilation and keeping house dust to a minimum through regular dusting and vacuuming. We can all streamline our line-ups of cleaning and personal grooming products and be more aware of the new consumer products we introduce into our homes. Other indoor environments that we spend a lot of time in include schools, offices and public transport. These are places where we have far less control over our immediate environment yet paradoxically where much more utilitarian product choices are often made. Often a lot of cheaper, more synthetic, stain and flame-resistant building products are used. In some cases, the toxic combinations are so bad that the place is said to have sick building syndrome – a phenomenon whereby the general health of a high proportion of the people who work in it is adversely affected. Changing the chemical content of these places is far more difficult than changing things at home, but the same simple solutions apply – plenty of ventilation and dust removal. And if you really think you or your kids are suffering from your exposure to toxic chemicals at work or school, do some-thing about it. Discuss it with fellow workers or parents and take it up with the powers that be. No one should have to work or be educated in a significantly polluted environment.

5

Rules and regulations

"Contemporary civilization differs in one particularly distinctive feature from those which preceded it: speed. The change has come about within a generation" – noted the historian Marc Bloch, writing in the nineteen-thirties. This observation certainly holds true for the synthetic chemicals industry and its relatively short, but extraordinarily prolific history. In the developed world, we now live as a generation of consumers who expect new and improved products on a weekly basis. We purchase gadgets, gizmo's, home comforts and everyday items without really thinking about what goes into them or where they go when we finish with them. Coming up close behind us are new mass markets such as China and India with almost unfathomable potential demand for chemically-laden consumer goods. Given what we know about rising rates of non-infectious diseases and pervasive global contaminants, one thing we should pass on to developing nations is the knowledge and support to instigate the best possible regulatory measures to control chemicals so that their manufacture and use is sustainable. But how do we do that when our own regulatory systems are in such a ragged, piecemeal and half-cocked state?

Regulation matters

The best way to sum up the brief history of chemicals legislation is that it has been reactionary – action being taken after a problem has been identified. This is different to the pharmaceutical industry where products are subject to much greater safety testing before they can be bought to market, and where regular updates occur as technology and medical practice evolve. Although it is a far from perfect industry and terrible mistakes like DES and thalidomide do occur, it's still a world away from the situation we find ourselves in with chemical industry regulation. The publication of 'Silent Spring' by Rachel Carson in 1962 acted as a wake up call to the world about the impact of synthetic chemicals on nature. Yet almost half a century later, the regulatory systems are still floundering in the face of a burgeoning chemical industry and past mistakes. Furthermore the fundamental difficulties in categorically testing or proving whether a chemical, alone or in combination with others, 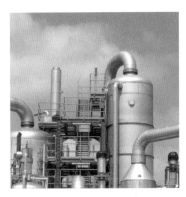 does harm or not remains elusive. Even though we now know beyond doubt about POPs and PBTs, other chemicals with similar hazard profiles are still being produced in high volumes and are added to products that we come into intimate contact with, without adequate testing and regulation.

The reactionary chemicals policy is clearly unsatisfactory, especially in view of the ever-increasing evidence of the role that synthetic substances play in many health issues, the sad and undeniable evidence of their widespread effects on wildlife, and the fact that there is probably not one single place on earth uncontaminated by man-made chemicals.

Many commentators on big business have remarked on the general systemic bias towards large, global operators when considering regulations that claim to protect the environment and public health. Although the regulatory regimes may be well-intentioned, they often fail. This is partly because of the 'revolving door' situation, where regulatory bodies hire past and future employees of the industries they are supposed to regulate. Then there is the fact that governments are always juggling the need to encourage industry to develop new products and processes, with desperate attempts to limit the potential harm. Even if it is not diluted through the intense lobbying efforts of regulated industries, legislation simply cannot keep up with the current pace of technological change and development. For example in the US, 1,000 new chemicals enter commercial markets every year while the National Toxicology Program (the agency responsible for assuring the safety of these chemicals) can only manage to conduct testing on around 25 of them annually – and even that's often not exhaustive.

A Brief History of Global Chemical Regulation

1962 – Many environmentalists would argue that the publication of **Rachel Carson's 'Silent Spring'** gave the impetus that launched the contemporary environmental movement

1983 – Brundtland Commission Report – The Brundtland report illustrated the widespread human concern for the state of the environment and popularised the phrase 'sustainable development'. This was defined as a way to meet 'the needs of the present without compromising the ability of future generations to meet their own needs'. There were two key issues: a) that development should not be just about bigger profits and higher standards of living for a minority – it should be about making life better for everyone and b) this should not involve destroying or recklessly using up our natural resources, nor should it involve polluting the environment

1992 – The Rio 'Earth Summit' Declaration on Environment and Development was key, from a chemicals regulation point of view, because Chapter 19 addressed the environmentally-sound management of toxic chemicals including the prevention of illegal international traffic in toxic and dangerous products. Additionally, in the declaration itself Principle 15 stated: 'In order to protect the environment, the precautionary approach shall be widely applied by States according to their capabilities. Where there are threats of serious or irreversible damage, lack of full scientific certainty shall not be used as a reason for postponing cost-effective measures to prevent environmental degradation'. This was where the Precautionary Principle was first given legal credence, giving the environment the benefit of the doubt over unsustainable development

2001 – UN POPs convention – 'The 2001 Stockholm Convention on persistent organic pollutants (POPs)' is one of the major achievements in global chemicals regulation and led directly on from the Earth Summit Chapter 19 and the Declaration Principles from Rio. Signatories agreed to phase out and limit production of 12 POPs – PBT chemicals that can cause biological havoc. The treaty also outlined key principles for a less toxic world including the prevention of new toxic, persistent, and bioaccumulative chemicals; reduction of existing ones; and substitution with less dangerous alternatives. At present, however, the Stockholm Treaty covers only 12 chemicals: nine pesticides, polychlorinated biphenyls (PCBs), and the industrial by-products dioxins and furans. Brominated Flame Retardants and Perfluorinates are up for consideration for POP status:- if this were to occur it would mean radical changes for the chemicals industry.

The UN should be commended for the POPs convention, so too those nations that played a key role and made sure that it came to fruition. But it does only address 12 compounds, many of which had already been banned in developed nations like the UK, other EU nations and the US and Canada since the 1970s. A more sceptical view could ask what took responsible governments so long, nearly 40 years, to try to get global controls on such damaging substances? And what about the rest of the chemicals that are manufactured, traded and used in consumer products? In the EU this number is believed to be about 30,000 chemicals. How well are those being regulated? The answer is very poorly.

Not only has the EU tried and failed to regulate chemicals adequately, so too has the US. While both have tried to implement more stringent testing on new substances coming onto the market, old substances that have been around for a long time are still allowed to be used despite little or no safety data. It is that 'burden of the past', all those substances that have been developed over time about which we know so little, that are of great concern. Any responsible society would say don't use a chemical until you have tested it adequately enough to know that it is safe for humans and wildlife. Industry's response is very different. Their message is along the lines of, we have used these chemicals for decades, there are no obvious negative effects, so let us carry on using them without testing them. But, as this book reveals, such confidence is misplaced. How can a manufacturer of a chemical or compound, without adequate testing, convince you, the consumer, that their substance is not a contributory factor in decreasing fertility, the increasing number of birth defects or rising incidences of diabetes and various cancers? Without any data, we can say that certain diseases are increasing but we cannot say why.

It is against this global backdrop that the **EU decided that a new chemicals regime was needed**. When the UK held Presidency of EU in 1998, it said that new chemicals legislation should:

- address the knowledge gap on the tens of thousands of substances on the market in consumer products to which humans, wildlife and the wider environment are exposed constantly ie. to address the burden of the past

- reverse the burden of proof to make chemical companies do sufficient testing to make sure the chemical is safe before it goes on the market – rather than make it the responsibility of the regulator.

Following on from this the EU Commission wrote the '*Chemicals White Paper*' and this lead to REACH.

REACH – Regulation, Evaluation and Authorisation of Chemicals.

REACH is a proposal for a major new system to test a large number of chemicals for their effects on human health and the environment (ie. to supply adequate safety data on the chemicals that we have been using 'blind' for decades) plus a reversal of burden of proof – where 'no data, no market' is the rule, not the exception. So if a company doesn't have the data to say a chemical it produces is safe then it will get taken off the market.

The key aim of REACH is to protect humans, wildlife and the environment from chemical harm whilst not undermining the competitiveness of EU chemical manufacturing. From a consumer point of view, within REACH there are key elements that, if enforced, should protect consumers and the wider environment and these are what the environmental NGOs like WWF, FOE and Greenpeace want to see delivered.

These key elements are:

- **To stop the use of chemicals that are of very high concern** ie. chemicals that are persistent, bioaccumulative and toxic (PBTs), very persistent and very bioaccumulative chemicals VPVBs and endocrine-disrupting chemicals (EDCs) where human, wildlife or wider environmental exposure can occur

- **Substitution** – chemicals that contaminate the environment should be replaced with safer, less toxic alternatives

- **The Right To Know (RTK)** – where manufacturers and consumers have a right to know which chemicals are in what products

- **Reversal of the burden of proof** from the regulators to the manufacturers and distributors

- **No data no market** ie. if a manufacturer does not have the safety data for a chemical it should not be used in consumer products.

So, will it REACH the parts other legislation has failed to?

In its first incarnation the REACH proposal was expected to make dramatic improvements to chemical industry legislation and to cause a major shake-up in accountability within the industry-leading to extensive testing on 30,000 economically traded chemicals in the EU. The EU predicted that the successful implementation of REACH would bring savings in healthcare of over 50 billion Euros over a 30 year period. However, after what some EU officials claim to be the biggest lobbying effort they have ever seen, from European and American chemical manufacturers, the testing requirements have been diluted by two thirds and further loopholes are expected to be revealed as the intense lobbying pressure is maintained. Particularly worrying is the component addressing EDCs. How much proof will be needed before countries within the EU stop the most vulnerable members of our society (babies and children) being exposed to such worrying chemicals. Many people object to this American-style, stunt-and-favours type of pressure and think it's time for the regulation-hungry EU to start regulating the lobbyists.

So what can we expect?

Reducing our dependency on common toxic chemicals requires a combination of factors, ideally, all happening to be working together at the same time.

These include:

• strong laws binding industrial commitment to innovation

• greater public awareness and consumer participation in the demand for toxic-free products and processes

• In the absence of strong precautionary laws, product labelling systems are especially important since they can help to extend the public's right-to-know about toxic materials used in consumer products, thereby empowering consumers to refuse to buy products containing particular toxic chemicals. Labelling systems are already in use for a number of products, including PVC-free toys, mercury-free thermometers, organically grown cotton T-shirts, and chlorine-free bleached paper. In the short term probably the best we can realistically expect is better labelling and the gradual phasing out of known PBT chemicals. What we cannot expect is a sudden generalised precautionary approach to be adopted by an industry that has gone unchecked and virtually unregulated for many, many decades. The REACH legislation exemplifies 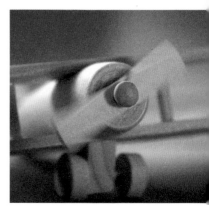 the ways in which lobbying has become at once a refined and a behind-closed-doors political tool. Following the American example, lobbying is a key tool of big business to enable it to have its own way, and its way is maximisation of profits, not the health of the nation.

Without wanting to paint too dark a picture, the reality is that the chance of the industry pulling itself up by its green boot-strings in the near future, without intense consumer and regulatory pressure, is a long shot from a pea shooter. While regulation attempts are admirable and every step forward should be acknowledged and applauded, the overriding concern is that enforcing any regulation on such a disparate, prolific and powerful industry takes such a long time, and there's a new generation on the way now. It should be enough to know that, most likely without exception, (but since we haven't tested everyone on the planet we have to say that) every pregnant and lactating woman who exists on the earth today will, often unwittingly and certainly unwillingly, be exposing her unborn or new born child to a variety of chemicals. Many of these will be known to be toxic, most unknown whether they are or not, and there's not a damn thing she can do about it. This is unacceptable in any civilised society and as consumers we must stop blind sighting ourselves. We must ask, what makes this fabric 'crease-proof', this cleaner 'super-powered', this carpet 'stain-proof'? What mass of plastic, electronics and chemicals am I adding to global toxic waste every time I upgrade my phone, ipod, laptop, car etc? Most importantly, what effect is all of our ignorance having on our children? We are all living in debt in more ways than one.

6

Some conclusions and observations

Health and fitness literature feeds us with the idea that we can de-tox, re-tox, and then de-tox again almost ad infinitum and at will. To a limited extent, with respect to many of the things that we knowingly and consensually do, a period of healthy eating, exercise, staying off drink, drugs and cigarettes will allow the body time to expel built up accumulated toxicity. However, as we have seen, when it comes to certain classes of toxic chemicals the 'pollution' can be very long-term and almost irreversible. With cruel irony, short of having a baby, it can be argued that it's very difficult to reduce the PBT chemicals that accumulate in the body's tissues.

Novel molecular constructions might offer up new ways to fry our eggs but unfortunately we now have to ask ourselves: what's in the egg I'm frying in the first place, what was in the chicken that gave rise to the egg and what's in the pan I'm frying it in? It might be the case that the chemical that makes frying your eggs easier could react with a chemical that has already bioaccumulated in the egg itself. When you eat the egg, it might bioaccumulate in you, then it may have a negative effect on your reproductive system, on your own eggs, or sperm. You could then pass this on to your offspring – and the old story about the chicken and the egg starts to take on a new and much more sinister meaning.

Another ominous upshot, from research carried out on endocrine-disrupting chemicals, indicates that they seem to be hitting the male of the species particularly hard and specifically in their (increasingly un-descended) testicles. It could be because more research has been carried out on the 'feminising' effects of certain chemicals, but hypothetically, the combination of higher incidences of reproductive system birth defects in baby boys, lower sperm rates and rising cases of testicular cancer amongst young men could result in a steady de-masculinisation of the world. Put another way this could mean a gradual femi-nising of the world unwittingly brought about by the actions of corporations on

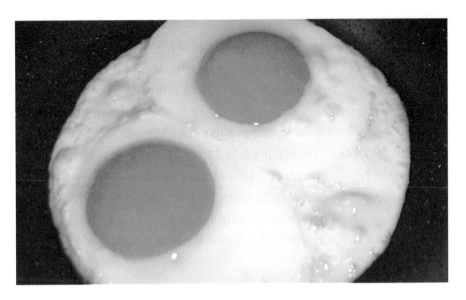

a generation of men-folk whose testicles and penises are shrinking, sexual potency deteriorating and ability to reproduce declining. A twisted feminist dream or natural selection with a chemical twist – who knows? What we do know is that we need sustainable or greener chemistry to be the rule not the exception. Adopting a precautionary policy when it comes to the use of new and old synthetic chemicals in consumer products is the only sensible way forward. We must give babies and children the benefit of the doubt and ensure adequate testing occurs, rather than continuing to use chemicals about which we do not have adequate knowledge.

But wait, the no-nonsense brigade chorus, we are all living longer so what's the big fuss about? Firstly 'we' is a very general term, and while average life expectancy may be increasing, a lot of us are living longer, but with various complaints that we weren't living with fifty years ago. Furthermore, there is the view that diabetes might be the first disease in decades to cause an overall decrease in life expectancy in the UK – and although childhood obesity generally gets the blame there is also research linking the rising rate of diabetes to exposure to toxic chemicals. Also, the problems posed by toxic chemicals are often more far-reaching and subtle than life-threatening conditions – it's about disruption of human and animal behaviour and the basic human right to be able to fulfil one's potential without attention deficit disorders, neurological impairments, messed-up hormones or the psychosexual burden of being born with ambiguous or deformed genitalia.

Taking endocrine-disrupting chemicals alone – hormones are the natural chemical messengers of life on earth – they tell squirrels when to hibernate, salmon when to swim upriver to spawn; they control when women ovulate plus a myriad of other essential human functions. They are present in the blood in minuscule concentrations and often for only short periods of time and yet have powerful effects on us. Witness mood-swinging adolescence, the power of adrenaline, sexual desire, PMT and male aggression – its hard enough keeping ourselves in check without fake messages flooding our systems. But as we've seen, many synthesised chemicals have been shown to be good imitators of our natural hormones, and some can actually interfere with this delicate, powerful, complex and intensely interrelated system. There is plenty of evidence of strange things afoot in wildlife – aquatic, avian and terrestrial – and since what we do to the animals we do to ourselves, the unavoidable, and distinctly unpalatable, truth is that it may already be starting to happen to us. One has to ask oneself how serious do things have to get before we collectively take action?

The risk assessment for chemicals added to everyday products is not like a risk assessment you would choose for yourself or those dependent on you. Would you say to yourself – I'll keep using this cream on my baby until it is proven to give my child a persistent behavioural disorder that may well affect her/his educational potential and social development. Of course not – you'd choose an alternative that you know is safe until the cream has been proven to have no short-mid-or-long-term effects. So, before you pop out for a few cocktails, think about the one you are slathering, massaging, slicking and spraying onto all the different parts of your body, the shampoos, body washes, nail varnishes, lipsticks, face creams, perfumes, aftershaves, shaving gels, hair gels, sprays, mousses' – you've probably got a whole range. None of us want to look like a raw faced monk who's personal care regime consists of a bit of old soap and a rough towel but we assure you, you can be pampered, soothed, and primped WITHOUT poisoning yourself. Choose products that don't have petroleum by-products in them, choose greener, cleaner options, ideally without parabens, formaldehyde, phthalates et al. Chemical solutions for consumer products are generally mass

116

market and designed to make easy living cheap but there may be a heavy personal cost as well as the obvious environmental one. If you thought that the synthetic musk in your aftershave might have a negative affect on your sperm count how attractive would it make you feel as you splashed it all over?

The major problem in all this is linking exposure to specific chemicals with specific illnesses because of the multiplicity of influences we are exposed to in contemporary life – let alone linking specific chemicals to factors such as effects on IQ, behaviour or immune system function. Yet where specific and tragic chemical accidents have occurred, there have been clear resultant effects on local populations, or, in the case of accidents like DES, on the offspring of the women prescribed it. This is all very compelling evidence for the precautionary approach to chemicals because laws take a long time to come into force. Look how long it took to make the case for cigarettes and cancer. Even with clear evidence, people are still, unwillingly, passively exposed to cigarette smoke and it is still legal for adults to puff their lungs out in rooms that children are in. The issue of synthetic chemicals, given their sheer quantity and ubiquity in consumer products, at first seems insurmountable. However, it has largely been a lack of scientific knowledge that has permitted what could be seen as greedy industry practice to have proceeded in the past with so little constraint and caution. The tobacco industry had the advantage of an addicted consumer on its side who simply didn't want to believe that their habit could possibly be the agent of their own deterioration. No one, as far as we know, is addicted to any of the toxic chemicals written about in this book – with the exception of rare and odd cases of addiction to certain perfumes. While some of us might reluctantly part company with the promise of a chemical company's fifties advertising slogan: 'Better things for better living....through chemistry', in the face of what's really at stake – the legacy that this leaves to our children and to the generation after them, the attachment seems a bit trite.

Also, although we often don't, we should all think about the broader and longer-term consequences of how we live. The phenomenon of global distillation (whereby the global winds of the world blow outwards from the hot equator to the two polar cold environments) combined with the sheer near-indestructible persistence of certain toxic chemicals means that many of them end up settling in the two far poles of the world. Thirty years ago, the most surprising fact known about the polar bear was that it could be quite aggressive – but now, sadly, it is that it is one of the most toxic animals on earth despite living far away from the sources of the industry that produces the substances that contaminate it. This is true of hundreds of contaminated animal populations, from fish to herring gulls, frogs to whales, and ultimately us.

There has to be a fundamental paradigm shift in the way we live with chemicals, especially now as the dawn of nano-technology brings with it a new type of potentially even more invasive agent in the form of new nano-toxic substances where smaller particles of previously harmless substances start to make it to places they've never been before.

"Nanotechnology is likely to be particularly important in the developing world, because it involves little labour, land or maintenance; it is highly productive and inexpensive; and it requires only modest amounts of materials and energy."

From *Innovation: applying knowledge in development*, report of the UN Millennium Project, Task force on Science, Technology and Innovation, 2005

Nano-particles are tiny (less than 100nm) and are already used in products as diverse as anti-aging creams, sunscreens, anti-bacterial socks and tennis racquets. They are touted as 'miracle molecules' and nano-technology is increasingly used in new pharmaceuticals and medical applications. For example, the headline-grabbing breast cancer drug Herceptin has a nano-sized antibody that can infiltrate the HER 2 receptors of tumour cells and tell them to stop growing. The potential for nano-technology to help treat cancer and other medical conditions is clearly very exciting. Their use in sunscreens and cosmetics, on the other hand, is arguably quite superfluous in the light of early research indicating that certain nano-particle chemicals can be very toxic, especially when in water (shown to cause rapid onset brain damage in fish and to kill water fleas living in water contaminated with 'bucky balls' – a particular kind of nano-particle). Since many nano-particles can cross the blood/brain barrier in humans, precaution is, you might say, a no-brainer. If any doubt exists over their potential toxicity to the environment, to wildlife and to us, then a lot more research needs to be

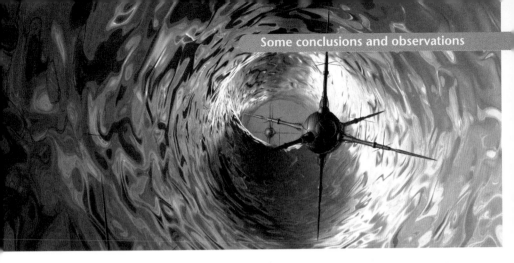

undertaken before the chemical industry should be allowed to harness their extraordinary powers to imbue new and improved status to a whole range of consumer products. The market for nano-particles will approach one billion dollars in 2007, yet neither government regulations nor labelling requirements exist in any country currently.

We're just coming round from the turn of the 21st century to see that we are the generation that is both waving and drowning. We know beyond doubt that irre-versible damage is being done to the earth's eco-systems and while we might make personal decisions to drive our cars less or stop smoking, our planet is still smouldering in front of our eyes. We know exactly how to change the ways of the world for a sustainable future, but don't – like the insatiable alcoholic we are on the brink of disaster and so we get even more loaded. It's an appalling lack of environmental responsibility fuelled by bossy litigious corporations and a consumer culture based on ease and disposability. There is no apparent limit to human invention and it is only natural to want to drive new cars, have foreign holidays and use mobile phones, but we need to rethink collectively how we do this so that we behave more sustainably. Against this background, self-education is essential – the head-in-the-sand option cannot exist. It is the authors' personal viewpoint that once people know a little bit about many of the everyday chem-icals used in consumer products, they will see that the only sensible choice they can make is to try to avoid them. We do. It might appear daunting at first, but with some simple everyday actions it is possible to dramatically reduce exposure to common toxic chemicals – and consumers have power – so challenge your local MPs, retailers and manufacturers – ask questions and demand answers!

119

TOXIC AVOIDANCE TIPS

1 Ventilate your home and other indoor environments

2 Dust and vacuum (with a well-sealed unit) your home regularly

3 Avoid soft plastics

4 Avoid synthetic fragrance

5 Streamline your personal care range of products and choose organic, fragrance-free, petrochemical-free options wherever possible

6 Don't buy dry-clean-only clothes

7 Choose natural floorings over synthetic where possible

8 Avoid products infused with brominated flame retardants

9 Avoid non-stick cookware

10 Avoid stain repellents

11 Avoid easy-iron clothing

12 Avoid fungicide-treated socks, shoes or other clothing

13 Avoid plastic food boxes

12 Don't microwave in plastic

Become label savvy – know what to look out for and avoid **13**

Be aware of the VOC levels and other chemicals in DIY products and always heed safety instructions **14**

Use herbal remedies for your pets flea infestations **15**

Use herbal remedies for head lice infestations in children **16**

Preparing as much of your diet as possible from fresh ingredients helps to avoid the plethora of chemicals used in food processing and packaging **17**

Educate yourself, demand greener alternatives **18**

Ask local authorities how they control weeds in parks and on school playing fields **19**

Query the chemical content of products you are suspicious about with the manufacturer or retailer **20**

Discuss the issue of toxic chemicals in consumer products with other people – word of mouth has always been the best form of PR and the more people know and talk about these issues the more pressure ultimately is bought to bear on the regulators and the industry they are supposed to regulate. **21**

Glossary of terms used in The toxic consumer

AHTN	6-Acetyl-1,1,2,4,4,7-hexamethyltetraline
BFR	Brominated flame retardant
BPA or BpA	Bisphenol A
DEA	(cocamide) diethanolamine
Deca BDE	Deca-brominated diphenyl ether
DDT	Dichloro-diphenyl-trichloroethane
DEHP	Di(2-ethylhexyl) phthalate
DES	Diethylstilbestrol
EDC	Endocrine-disrupting chemical
EDTA	Ethylenediaminetetraacetic acid
FD&C	United States Federal Food, Drug, and Cosmetic Act
GNP	Gross national product
HHCB	(1,3,4,6,7,8-hexahydro-4,6,6,7,8,8-hexamethylcy-clopenta- -2-benzopyran and related isomers)
MCS	Multiple chemical sensitivity
MDF	Medium density fibreboard
MIT	Methylisothiazolinone
Octa BDE	Octa-brominated diphenyl ether
PAH	Polycyclic aromatic hydrocarbons

PBDE	Poly-brominated diphenyl ether
PBT	Persistent bioaccumulative and toxic
PCB	Polychlorinated biphenyl
Penta BDE	Penta-brominated diphenyl ether
PERC	Perchloro ethylene
PFC	Perfluorinated chemical
PFOA	Perfluorooctanoic acid
PFOS	Perfluorooctane sulfonate
POP	Persistent organic pollutant
PVC	Poly-vinyl chloride
REACH	Regulation, Evaluation and Authorisation of Chemicals
RTK	Right To Know
SLS	Sodium lauryl sulphate
TBT	Tributyltin
TDS	Testicular dysgenesis syndrome
USEPA	United States Environmental Protection Agency
VOC	Volatile organic compound
VPVB	Very persistent, very bioaccumulative

Bibliography

Books

Baillie-Hamilton, Paula. (Jan 2005). *Stop the 21st Century Killing You: Toxic Chemicals Have Invaded Our Life. Fight Back Eliminate Toxins, Tackle Illness, Get Healthy and LIve Longer.* Vermilio).

Rapp, Doris. (Oct 2003). *Our Toxic World – A Wake Up Call ,* (Practical Allergy Res Fndtn).

Johansen, Bruce E. (June 30, 2003). *The Dirty Dozen: Toxic Chemicals and the Earth's Future.* Praeger Publishers.

Colborn, Theo. Peterson Myers, John. Dumanoski, Diane. (March 1996). *Our Stolen Future: Are We Threatening Our Own Fertility, Intelligence and Survival? A Scientific Detective Story.* EP Dutton.

Bibliography

Organisations and Websites

WWF UK – www.wwf.org.uk/chemicals or www.detox.panda.org

Greenpeace – www.greenpeace.org.uk/products/toxics

FOE – www.foe.co.uk/campaigns/safer_chemicals

WEN – www.wen.org.uk

CHE – The Collaborate on Health and the Environment
– www.healthandenvironment.org

Rachel – www.rachel.org

Our Stolen Future – www.ourstolenfuture.org

EWG – www.ewg.org

Health-report.co.uk

European Commission – *DG Environment – responsible for REACH –*
http://ec.europa.eu/environment/chemicals/reach.htm

DEFRA – *Chemicals Unit – responsible for REACH in UK –*
www.defra.gov.uk/environment/chemicals/reach/index.htm

CIA – *UK Chemical Industry Association –* www.cia.org.uk

ES&T – *Environmental Science and Technology - journal –*
– http://pubs.acs.org/journals/esthag/index.html

EHP – *Environmental Health Perspectives - journal –* www.ehponline.org

Reference Index

Chapter 1

1 IPCS Global Assessment on the State of the Science of Endocrine Disruptors, WHO, 2002. Janssen S, Solomon G, Schettler T. (2005). Chemical Contaminants and Human Disease: A summary of Evidence by CHE, USA. Birnbaum LS, Fenton SE. (2003). Cancer and developmental exposure to endocrine disruptors. Environ Health Perspect. 2003 Apr;111(4):389-94. Clapp D, Howe G, Jacobs Lefevre M. (2005). Environmental and Occupational Causes of Cancer: A review of Recent Scientific Literature. (2005). Lowell Centre for Sustainable Production, University of Massachusetts, USA.

Chapter2

2 Birnbaum Staskal D. (2004). Brominated Flame Retardants: Cause for Concern? Env Health Persp, vol 112, 2004.

3 Mothers' Milk: Record Levels of Fire Retardants Found in American Mothers' Breast Milk. Part 3: Health Risks of PBDEs. 2006. Environmental Working Group, USA.

4 1.SAB (2006) Science Advisory Board review of the EPA's draft risk assessment of potential human health effects associated with PFOA and its salts. 30 May 2006.EPA-SAB-06-006. US EPA, Washington. 2.OECD 2002 Environment Directorate Joint Meeting of the Chemicals Committee and the Working Party on Chemicals, Pesticides and Biotechnology. Co-operation on Existing Chemicals Hazard Assessment of Perfluorooctoane Sulfonate (PFOS) and its Salts. ENV/JM/RD(2002)17/FINAL. 21 Nov 2002 3.Keml 2004. Dossier in support for a nomination of PFOS to the UN-ECE LRTAP Protocol and the Stockholm Convention.

5 Sharpe R, Irvine S. (2004). How Strong is the Evidence of a Link Between Environmental Chemicals and Adverse Effects on Human Reproductive Health? BMJ, vol 328 447-451. Fisher J. (2004). Environmental Anti-androgens and Male Reproductive Health: Focus on Phthalates and Testicular Dysgenesis Syndrome. Reproduction (2004) 127 305-315

6 Munoz-de-Toro M, Markey C, Wadia PR, Luque EH, Rubin BS, Sonnenschein C, Soto AM. 2005. Perinatal exposure to bisphenol A alters peripubertal mammary gland development in mice. Endocrinology. Sep;146(9):4138-47.), male reproductive system defects (Vom Saal FS, Hughes C. An extensive new literature concerning low-dose effects of Bisphenol a shows the need for a new risk assessment.Environ Health Perspect. 2005 Aug;113(8):926-3), miscarriage (Sugiura-Ogasawara M, Ozaki Y, Sonta S, Makino T, Suzumori K. 2005. Exposure to bisphenol A is associated with recurrent miscarriage.Hum Reprod.Aug;20(8):2325-9.), immune system defects (Yoshino S, Yamaki K, Li X, Sai T, Yanagisawa R, Takano H, Taneda S, Hayashi H, Mori Y. (2004). Prenatal exposure to bisphenol A up-regulates immune responses, including T helper 1 and T helper 2 responses, in mice. Immunology Jul;112(3):489-95. Alizadeh M, Ota F, Hosoi K, Kato M, Sakai T, Satter MA.2006. Altered allergic cytokine and antibody response in mice treated with bisphenol A. J Med Invest. 2006 Feb;53(1-2):70-80.), polycystic ovarian disease (Takeuchi T, Tsutsumi O, Ikezuki Y, Takai Y, Taketani Y.2004. Positive relationship between androgen and the endocrine disruptor, bisphenol A, in normal women and women with ovarian dysfunction. Endocr J. Apr;51(2): 165-9.), and recent research has even revealed a possible link to obesity (Masuno, H, T Kidani, K Sekiya, K Sakayama, T Shiosaka, H Yamamoto and K Honda. 2002. bisphenol A in combination with insulin can accelerate the conversion of 3T3-L1 fibroblasts to adipocytes. Journal of Lipid Research 3:676-684.), insulin resistance and diabetes (Alonso-Magdalena, P, Morimoto S, Ripoll C, Fuentes E, Nadal A, 2006. The Estrogenic Effect of Bisphenol-A Disrupts the Pancreatic ß-Cell Function in vivo and Induces Insulin Resistance. Environmental Health Perspectives 114:106-112.

Also available from Impact Publishing

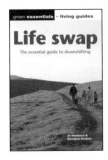

Life swap
– The essential guide to downshifting

Fed up with your current life? Spending too much and enjoying too little? Trapped in a stressful cycle of work and commitments? *Life Swap* shows you that there is an alternative – and if you care enough it is achievable. We give you the full low-down on the emotional and financial traps, the psychology for success, the money issues, work/life balance and the trick to changing your habits and expectations.

ISBN: 1 904601 43 X   **£7.99**

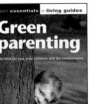

Green parenting
– Choosing what's best for you, your child and the environment

Lifestyle choices will influence how our children grow up – so what part should the consideration of health issues, organic living and the environment play when we bring up children?

Green Parenting takes you on a practical step-by-step journey from pregnancy through birth and babies, to toddlers and teenagers, offering advice you can act on now. When even small changes can make a big difference to you and your children, this practical guide will prove invaluable.

ISBN: 1 904601 39 1   **£7.99**

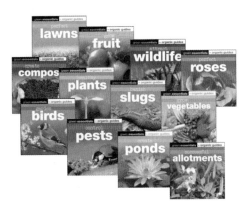

Green Essentials
– organic gardening guides

Practical, fun and each one is focused on just one topic – making it the ideal way for busy gardeners or beginners to get all the top organic tips they need.

These books may be small but they're already making a big impression! And you know you can trust the organic advice they contain – all books carry the logos of Garden Organic (HDRA) and the Soil Association.

£2.99 each

www.impactpublishing.co.uk